# SHAPE-UP SHORTCUTS

*Kelly Jean*

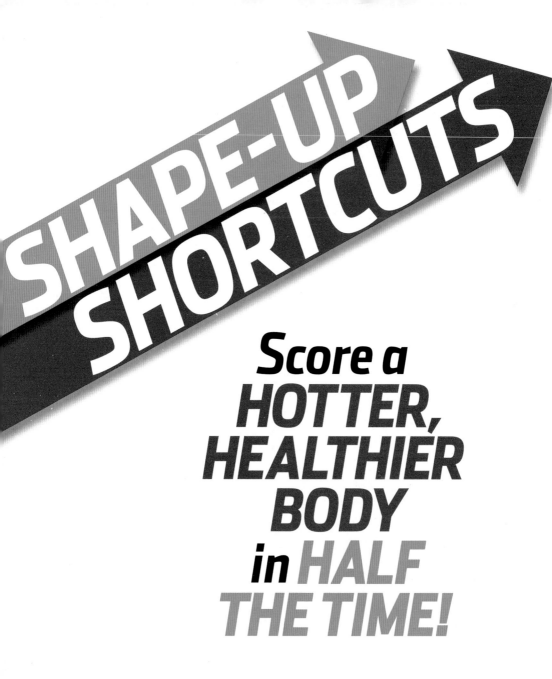

# SHAPE-UP SHORTCUTS

## Score a HOTTER, HEALTHIER BODY in HALF THE TIME!

Jen Ator, CSCS, and the editors of Women'sHealth®

RODALE

© 2013 by Rodale Inc.
Photographs © 2013 by Rodale Inc.

Rodale books may be purchased for business or promotional use or for special sales. For information, please write to: Special Markets Department, Rodale Inc., 733 Third Avenue, New York, NY 10017

*Women's Health* is a registered trademark of Rodale Inc.

Printed in the United States of America
Rodale Inc. makes every effort to use acid-free ∞, recycled paper ♻.

Book design by Mike Smith
Photographs by Beth Bischoff

Library of Congress Cataloging-in-Publication Data is on file with the publisher.

ISBN 978-1-62336-204-1 direct hardcover
ISBN 978-1-62336-203-4 trade paperback

Distributed to the trade by Macmillan

2 4 6 8 10 9 7 5 3 1 direct hardcover

2 4 6 8 10 9 7 5 3 1 trade paperback

We inspire and enable people to improve their lives and the world around them.
**rodalebooks.com**

No success is ever just about a finish line—it's about the people who are there for you every step of the race, cheering you on, picking you up, and making you feel like a winner regardless of the final score.
To my amazing family and friends . . .
thank you for being there to share in every accomplishment, big and small.

# CONTENTS

## PART I: SMALL CHANGES, BIG RESULTS

CHAPTER 1:
### THE SHORTCUT SECRET 
*Scoring a leaner, healthier body has never been this easy*

CHAPTER 2:
*Painless tips for reinventing your relationship with food*

CHAPTER 3:
*Spend less time in the gym—and fast-track your results*

## PART II: GET FIT—FAST!

CHAPTER 4:
*The easiest fat-loss plan ever!*

CHAPTER 5:
*Turbocharge your metabolism and get lean fast*

# PART III: SHORTCUT SOLUTIONS

# ACKNOWLEDGMENTS

*Shape-Up Shortcuts* would not have been possible without the help of so many. I'd like to take this opportunity to thank a few of them.

Michele Promaulayko: I'll be forever grateful that you welcomed me onto the *Women's Health* team more than 4 years ago and for your continued support, trust, and guidance. It's been an honor to work for such a game-changing brand, and I can't wait to see what's next for us.

Adam Campbell: You have been a mentor, friend, and an invaluable bank of knowledge. I couldn't have dreamed that I would be here today, and I can say with no exaggeration that without your time and attention over the years, I wouldn't be.

I'd especially like to thank Maria Rodale and the entire Rodale family for spearheading the passionate company that makes this all possible; Mary Ann Naples, Amy King, Jeff Csatari, Debbie McHugh, Ursula Cary, Mike Smith, Hope Clarke, Jess Fromm, and the rest of the books team for this incredible opportunity and for their tremendous efforts that made it a reality; Michelle Janowitz for her careful copyediting; Beth Bischoff for her beautiful photography; Melissa Wood, Lauren Williams, and Devon Ericksen for being amazing "models" of health, fitness, and happiness; Lindsey Benoit and Allison Keane, in advance, for their tireless promotion of this book; Theresa Griggs, Cathryne Keller, Genevieve Nutting, and especially Caitlin Carlson, for their invaluable behind-the-scenes work. This book is only possible thanks to each of you.

To the entire *Women's Health* staff: I'm truly privileged to work beside such intelligent, supportive, and talented women. This is my dream job, in no small part thanks to all of you.

Fitness is a deep-rooted foundation in my life, and I have had so many influential coaches, teammates, and mentors. (Like Jen Haney: You always demanded our best effort—it has made me a better athlete and person.) But I'm truly indebted to the brilliant fitness experts who have been willing to share their unparalleled knowledge with me. Even at the top of their game, they never stop improving—which keeps me inspired and elevates the entire industry. In particular . . . Rachel Cosgrove: You have been an irreplaceable part of the *Women's Health* fitness team; we are stronger (literally!) because of you. Craig Ballantyne, Mike Boyle, Hannah Davis, Todd Durkin, BJ Gaddour, Tony Gentilcore, Bill Hartman, David Jack, Andrew Kastor, Robert dos Remedios, Mike Robertson, Dan Trink (and Joe Dowdell and everyone at Peak Performance), Mark Verstegen, and Valerie Waters: I'm humbled by your enthusiastic support and honored by your contributions— within these pages and over the years in *Women's Health*.

Grandma: You've used every birthday, Halloween, Easter, Valentine's Day, and just-because opportunity to fill my mailbox. In an age of text, Facebook, and gchat, you remind me that some shortcuts aren't worth taking—and nothing replaces the thoughtfulness of a handwritten note.

To my brothers: Tim, you support, love, and look out for me (especially when it comes to my music choices)—what more could I ask for in a big brother? Kyle, I don't know what our family would have done without you; keep working hard on and off the field—and always save Christmas Eve for cookie deliveries.

Mom: You gave this small-town Ohio girl the confidence to chase her wildest dreams (like working for a major women's magazine in New York City) and taught her to take pride in being smart, strong, and driven. I'm a more ambitious and grateful person through your example.

Dad: You've put in endless miles to make my dreams come true. Thank you for showing up to every single game, no matter what. The sidelines have changed (you check my tweets instead of my stats), but you've never stopped rooting for me. Your advice continues to push me: Walk it off, stay positive, and dig deep for one more "Sprint!"

# Your Dream Body Starts Here

## "I just don't have time. . . ."

It's one of the most turned-to excuses for not working out—and it's not entirely inaccurate. Sure, most of us could spend fewer minutes surfing Facebook or catching up on episodes of *The Bachelor*, but even when you just consider the average person's must-do list (like sleeping, working, eating, commuting, showering—just to name a few), 24 hours sure do start to fill up fast.

Let's get something straight right out of the gate: I'm not here to challenge your time-crunched schedule—and I'm certainly not going to make you feel guilty for putting off a workout from time to time. *Fitness* is in my job title, and even I'm not immune to daily time-management (and motivation) struggles. I spend long hours behind a desk (and not a standing one). I work late, and I hardly ever get a full 8 hours of sleep. I actually enjoy and look forward to working out, and even I'm guilty of letting weeks pass without going to the gym. So trust me, my viewpoint comes from nowhere close to a high horse. I get where you're coming from, because I'm right there next to you.

Time (or lack of it) is an easy thing to blame, but the truth is that your schedule is not the biggest thing stopping you from feeling leaner, stronger, and more energized—it's your mentality.

That's bcause too many women fall into an all-or-nothing mind-set when it comes to diet and exercise. In a drive to see lightning-fast, jaw-dropping results, they seek out extremes; they spend hours at the gym, nix every "bad" food in the book, count every calorie, and allow very little room for error. In short, women assume that results demand perfection.

# "Every day is another chance to change your life."

—UNKNOWN

Unfortunately, in most cases—after a few days, weeks, or maybe months—this enthusiastic diligence slows—or worse, backfires—spiraling women back to the "nothing" end of the effort spectrum. They give up because the so-called rules of weight loss aren't realistic or sustainable.

That's because many of us focus on what we *can't* do. We can't make it to the gym for an hour every day; we can't give up our glass of wine at dinner; we can't learn to like vegetables; and we can't say no to chocolate. And because we see these things as weight-loss prerequisites, we compensate by saying, "I'll *try*." We say, "I'll give it a shot!"—I'll try to eat only salads for lunch, or make it to boot camp five times a week, or avoid all sweets—even though we know this ideal is flawed from the get-go. But no one said it better than Yoda (not even my dad, who has repeated it to me more times than I can possibly count): "No, try not. Do or do not—there is no try." At the end of the day, saying you'll try is just as good as saying you won't.

# "I can accept failure, everyone fails at something. But I can't accept not trying."

—MICHAEL JORDAN

But exercise, healthy eating, and losing weight don't
have to be such a burden. You don't—and I'd argue shouldn't—have to
feel like you're following a set of strict or severe rules. In fact, quite the
opposite: When you focus on doing things that are fast, easy, effective,
and, yes, even enjoyable, you're more likely to repeat them. It's the root
of what experts call the Self-Determination Theory, which boils down to
this: The more you do stuff you like to do (and not what you think you
should do), the more you'll keep doing it. The benefits of this intrinsic, or
internal, motivation have been proven in studies across the board—from
education to health care to parenting. In exercise research, intrinsically
motivated exercisers were more likely than those who were nagged by
friends or family to continue working out for 6 months or more.

At the heart of true long-term success is repetition. When you take
a look at the principal achievement among people who seem to always
be in phenomenal shape, you'll likely see a common denominator: They
have made being active and eating healthy a consistent part of their
way of life. It isn't a switch they turn on before beach season or a big
event, then shut off as soon as it's over. By following their lead, eventually what you eat and how much you move will become nearly uncon-
scious habits, rather than constant daily stressors. Instead of throwing
off your routine, you will find that these healthy decisions have become
an integral part of it.

This doesn't mean it will be any easier to find time, though. Researchers at the University of Alberta in Edmonton found that even for people
who love to exercise, scheduling regular workouts still can be a challenge. A few years ago, I was out to dinner in New York City with the
incredibly fit, active, and vibrant LaJean Lawson, PhD, a 63-year-old
exercise scientist. I asked her, "What's your secret to staying in such
great shape?" Her answer was simple: Identify your "basic threshold"
of fitness that is impossible to fail. Early on, Lawson decided she had to

claim an unrelenting identity as a fit person, and she needed to perform an intentional fitness activity daily. Her basic threshold: one pullup or two full pushups. So at the end of every day, whether she is sick, or traveling, or crazy with work deadlines, she still does one of those two things. It may not sound like much, but, in less than 15 seconds a day, it has enabled her to maintain a very long streak of being a continuously active person.

While I loved the philosophy and her inspiring attitude, I was skeptical; there was no way something so basic could work for me. "She probably is just super petite naturally, or has an unnaturally speedy metabolism," I thought. I might have doubted her theory, but I gave it a shot anyway. My first basic threshold: walking to and from work (about 25 minutes each way), rather than taking a cab or the subway. It didn't take long to notice that instead of feeling defeated for missing a spin class, I was proud that I kicked off my heels and hiked home— even if it was raining, snowing, or late. Was the effort comparable?

# "Motivation is what gets you started. Habit is what keeps you going."

—JIM ROHN

Of course not, but it helped shift my mind-set and make me feel like I was still on track.

Lawson's modest approach stuck with me, and I have repeatedly tested—and proved—its effectiveness. (Walking is now part of my normal daily routine.) Every few months I shake up that bare minimum: Sometimes I choose three simple exercises—upper body, lower body, and core—and do 15 reps of each before I hop in the shower in the morning, or I climb at least 10 total flights of stairs each day. Other times, I simply commit to spending 10 minutes on the foam roller before bed. These activities don't outweigh my workouts, but they help connect the dots in between missed sessions and breed confidence rather than frustration. As Lawson so perfectly told me, "In the end, being able to claim your identity as a 'fit person' is as much a state of *being* as it is a state of *doing*."

That's why I'm so excited about *Shape-Up Shortcuts*. So many of us have lost sight of what we *can* do, probably because we think it's inconsequential and can't possibly make a difference. I've been there. I've shared that all-or-nothing mindset. As a collegiate Division I athlete, my workouts were measured in hours, not minutes. I knew what it felt like to push myself to my absolute physical and mental limit—and I assumed that anything less was slacking off. Rather than fitting my workouts into my routine, my day-to-day schedule revolved around my weight training, conditioning, practice, or games. Then I graduated and hit the real world, and that acute dedication was immediately unsustainable. Priorities shifted. My timed mile or squat max didn't make me better at my job, and spending hours at the gym each weekday wasn't as valued by my bosses as it was by my former coaches. With the exception of weekends, the best I could do was scrounge together around 30 minutes a day to exercise—and, really, what good could that do?

Thankfully, I've now learned that those 30 minutes can be all you actually need to transform your body—and maintain it for the rest of your life. As you flip through the following pages, you'll find thousands of effective and efficient diet and workout solutions. These shortcuts are not driven by the goal of fast (often temporary and fluctuating) weight loss. They don't come attached with strict rules or impractical plans, and they're not based on the latest fad diet or workout craze. Best of all, they generate the results you want, without consuming all your free time (in fact, no workout in this book will take you more than 30 minutes). These strategies are practiced by the country's leading fitness experts, tested by the world's top researchers, and proven by everyday women like you and me. Some of the strategies maximize the precious (and few) minutes you have; others actually minimize your time commitment. You don't have to use them all at once, and you don't have to use all of them. It's not about changing your life to fit with a workout or diet plan. It's about choosing a plan that works best with your life.

Shape-Up Shortcuts is your guide to being a little bit better—not perfect—every day for the rest of your life. If you commit to making at least one change each day, I promise your life and your body will dramatically improve. You will look leaner, feel more energetic, and improve your overall fitness. You may not be able to avoid every daily stressor, but my hope is that this book can help make sure your diet and fitness routine isn't one of them.

# Here's What You'll Find Inside...

Look for these features throughout the book for hundreds of fast and effective shortcuts.

- **2-Second Life Changers:** The easiest, fastest solutions to a slimmer, healthier life

- **Simple Swaps:** Effortless substitutions that make a huge impact

- **Lighter Bites:** Tips for trimming calories while still enjoying your favorite foods

- **Shape-Up Setbacks:** Common weight-loss pitfalls—and practical strategies for how to avoid them

- **Slim-Down Secrets:** Tricks and tips for staying lean for life

- **Lightning-Fast Meals:** Throw together delicious, waist-slimming meals in minutes

- **Leftover Loves:** Easy ways to make your food taste just as good the second time around

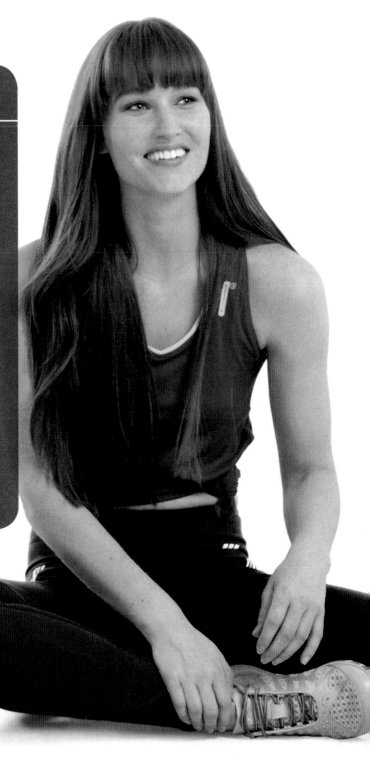

# PART I
## SMALL CHANGES, BIG RESULTS

### CHAPTER
# 01

# The
# Shortcut
# Secret

*Scoring a leaner, healthier body has never been this easy*

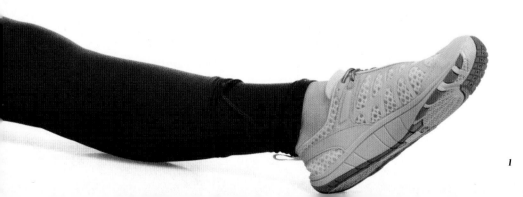

# Shortcut, noun

1. A route more direct than the one ordinarily taken
2. A means of saving time or effort
3. An accelerated way of doing something

When you hear the word *shortcut,* it may evoke a slightly negative connotation—one more or less interchangeable with cheating. Those who use shortcuts are cutting corners, taking the easy road, bypassing important steps, or being flat-out lazy. After all, we've all heard that "there are no shortcuts to any place worth going."

But when it comes to achieving a leaner, hotter, and healthier body, taking a more direct path can improve your success. That's because lasting and healthy weight loss isn't really as hard, complicated, or time consuming as it has always seemed, though you'd never know it—thanks to the revolving door of new diet and fitness crazes, each claiming to hold the key to the best-kept secret, which undoubtedly opposes at least a handful of other "revolutionary" plans.

All of this conflicting knowledge isn't making us smarter; it's just making it harder for the average person to figure out which road to take. It adds distraction and, all too often, unnecessary steps.

When you look at dieting through that lens, a shortcut might not sound all that terrible, right? That's where this book comes in—to help reduce the clutter, noise, and confusion so you can do less and get more out of it. As you'll start to realize, these shortcuts are actually only synonymous with one thing: *simplicity.*

# The First Step Toward Slim

⏩ According to a poll of nearly 6,300 people by the Institute for Medicine and Public Health at Vanderbilt University in Nashville, Tennessee, it's likely that you spend a stunning 56 hours a week sitting—staring at a computer screen, working the steering wheel, or collapsed in a heap in front of your high-def TV. And it turns out women may be more sedentary than men, since they tend to play fewer sports and hold less active jobs.

This downtime is now so prevalent that it has paved the road to a new area of medical study called inactivity physiology, which explores the effects of our increasingly butt-bound lives, as well as a deadly epidemic researchers have dubbed "sitting disease."

When muscles— especially the ones in your lower body—are immobile, circulation slows and you burn fewer calories. Key flab-burning enzymes responsible for breaking down triglycerides (a type of fat) simply start switching off. Sit for a full day and those fat burners plummet by 50 percent. The less you move, the less blood sugar your body uses; research shows that for every 2 hours spent on your backside per day, your chance of contracting diabetes goes up by 7 percent. Your risk for heart disease goes up too, because enzymes that keep blood fats in check are inactive. Inactivity can also raise hell on your posture and spine health: Your hip flexors and hamstrings shorten

 **2-SECOND LIFE CHANGER**

Each 10 percent rise in sedentary time is associated with a 3.1-centimeter larger waist circumference. Researchers found that the waist measurements of study participants who got up the most were more than 2 inches smaller than those of people who got up the least.

# THE PRICE OF CONVENIENCE

**Technological advances are awesome** for the most part, but in the past few decades they've sucked the "active" right out of living. Mayo Clinic researchers estimate that we burn 1,500 to 2,400 fewer calories per day than we did just 50 years ago. Here's a look at how the American woman's average weight has soared with the advent of modern conveniences.

| 1964 | 1967 | 1983 | 1994 | 2005 |
|------|------|------|------|------|
| Cable television reaches 1 million households | Amana introduces the home microwave oven | Apple introduces the first personal computers | Shopping malls arrive on the Web | 13 million people have BlackBerrys |
| 140 POUNDS | 144 POUNDS | 150 POUNDS | 152 POUNDS | 164 POUNDS |

and tighten, while the muscles that support your spine become weak and stiff. Not to mention, with less blood flow, fewer feel-good hormones are circulating to your brain, making you more prone to depression.

What's more, even if you exercise, you're not immune to these effects. We've become so sedentary that 30 minutes a day at the gym may not do enough to counteract the detrimental effects of 8, 9, or 10 hours of sitting. This is one big reason so many women still struggle with weight, blood sugar, and cholesterol woes despite keeping consistent workout routines. In fact, research has found that regardless of how much moderate to vigorous exercise a person does, those who take more breaks from sitting throughout the day have slimmer waists, lower BMIs (body mass indexes), and healthier fat and sugar levels in their blood than those who sit the most.

# Move a Little, Lose a Lot

▶ One of the most important and life-altering discoveries to come out of recent exercise research is that getting into shape isn't an all-or-nothing proposition. In fact, you can make a significant impact on your waistline without ever stepping foot in the gym.

Mayo Clinic researchers have extensively studied the impact of

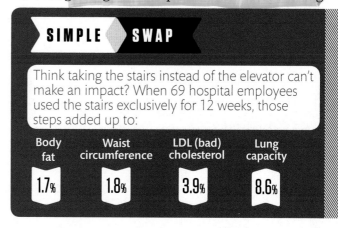

**SIMPLE SWAP**

Think taking the stairs instead of the elevator can't make an impact? When 69 hospital employees used the stairs exclusively for 12 weeks, those steps added up to:

| Body fat | Waist circumference | LDL (bad) cholesterol | Lung capacity |
|---|---|---|---|
| 1.7% | 1.8% | 3.9% | 8.6% |

activities like folding laundry, tapping your toes, standing up, even having sex—what they refer to as daily non-exercise activity thermogenesis (NEAT), or the energy you burn doing everything but exercise. They found that lean participants moved an average of 150 minutes more per day than the overweight participants—enough to burn 350 calories. A University of Missouri study found that staying on your feet blasts up to 60 calories more per hour than sitting. Adding these simple activities can help stave off the 1- to 2-pound weight gain most women accumulate every year—and it can keep your metabolism buzzing the way nature intended it to. Not to mention, getting off your butt for roughly an additional hour a day can decrease stress and heighten your mood, energy, focus, and productivity, reports the Centers for Disease Control and Prevention.

## # BY THE NUMBERS

**5.5** Number of years the average woman can add to her life expectancy if she is active in her free time.

Any amount of exercise is better than none, and research consistently proves that more frequent bursts of intense physical activity can produce the same muscle-building, fat-blasting, health-boosting benefits as the long-recommended 30 minutes a day. Studies have found that brief, vigorous workouts improve the body's ability to control blood sugar and lower blood pressure more than longer, less frequent sweat sessions; researchers in Denmark found that participants who completed shorter workouts burned more calories than those who logged more drawn-out ones.

What's more, the results seem to be cumulative, meaning you may get more points for repeated efforts—a set of squats in the morning, a brisk walk at lunch, and some pushups before bed—than for a marathon cardio session at the gym. And because a person can go all out

# BOUNCE BACK FASTER

If you take a few weeks or months (or even years!) off from exercise, you will most likely huff and puff and feel achy as your body gets back into the swing of things. But if you establish a history of regular exercise, your pain will be a lot more manageable. That's because any sweat equity you invest forges a cardiovascular and strength blueprint that helps you make gains faster and become less prone to soreness and injury.

It's a phenomenon aptly called "muscle memory." When you learn something new, whether it's how to do a split squat or snowboard, your brain fires up nerves that signal the muscle fibers to kick in. Once your muscle fibers get the memo from your brain to move, they start sending messages back. Movement activates sensors (called proprioceptors) in your muscles, tendons, and joints that constantly give feedback to your central nervous system about where your body is in space, so it knows what muscles to fire next. It's a continuous feedback loop from your brain to your muscles and back. Over time, your brain creates pathways through your central nervous system, and movements become automatic. That's why even if you haven't

hopped on a bike in years, your body remembers what to do.

Think of it like a health savings account: The earlier you start and the more you build, the better off you'll be later in life—even if your deposits stall for awhile. Case in point: Ohio University researchers put a group of women on a 2-day-a-week strength-training program for 20 weeks, and then let them lounge around for 8 months. When the researchers called these women back to the gym along with a group of women who'd never lifted before, they found that the previously trained group had retained most of their muscle memory. When they started pumping iron again, these women made gains more rapidly than the women with no history of strength training.

for 60 seconds but not 60 minutes, mini workouts can actually be more effective at sending your metabolism into overdrive, increasing your calorie burn during and after each fitness blast. Still not convinced? Here are seven ways short sweat sessions can improve your life.

## INCREASED STRENGTH

Just three 15-minute weight workouts a week can double a beginner's strength, report scientists at the University of Kansas. Not to mention, unlike the average person who quits a new program within a month, 96 percent of the study participants easily fit the short workouts into their lives.

## # BY THE NUMBERS

**20** Minutes of moderate to vigorous activity three to five times a week that has been shown to beat most other treatments for irritable bowel syndrome.

## DECREASED PERCEIVED EFFORT

If you think your workout is too hard, you're less likely to lose weight, reports the journal *Obesity*. When women were asked to rate how much a treadmill workout kicked their butts, those who ranked it the toughest packed on the most pounds a year later. The study's authors found that when you have a negative experience with exercise, you're less apt to do it.

## BLASTED BELLY FAT

In an Australian study, women who cranked out high-intensity interval training 3 days a week for 20 minutes (for 15 weeks) shed more fat than those who exercised for 40 minutes at a lower intensity over the same period.

# FIND YOUR STARTING LINE

I know what some of you might be thinking: If people aren't willing to dedicate an hour a day to their health and fitness goals, then they don't truly value them. A few of you may even be thinking that people looking for shortcuts don't deserve the same level of results as someone who put in more work. These are fair points. I agree that people will find time to prioritize the things that are most important to them.

But people also make time for the things they enjoy the most, as well; and I think that many people who allot an hour or more per day to, let's say, working out, are people who genuinely enjoy doing it. It goes beyond the fact that they value their health and their body—that time they find to work out is something they look forward to because it's an activity they truly like.

I'm in no way saying that long workouts and super-clean diets are bad or ineffective—I'm just saying you don't have to do them to get in great shape. The word to remember for lasting results is *consistency*. (To get better, it's *progress*.) Especially for beginners or those who seem to always fall off the wagon, the initial focus should be on learning simple exercise and nutrition tools and being consistent with them. To do this, starting with 10 minutes of exercise a day is a better idea than jumping straight into longer or tougher workouts. Over time, you may even learn to love it.

Look at this book as a starting place. The goal is to build lasting habits—not burn out. Once you've done that, by all means, progress! Challenge yourself to longer, tougher workouts. Hone your lean-eating patterns a little bit more. If at any time you fall off the wagon or hit a setback, come back to this book as a way of resetting and getting back on track.

## MANAGEABLE SCHEDULE

Previously inactive women who exercised four times a week gained just as much fitness in 16 weeks as those who did six workouts a week. What's more, they actually burned more total calories each day, reports a new study in the journal *Medicine & Science in Sports & Exercise*. What gives? Those who exercised more complained about not having enough time to get everything done—therefore, they were more likely to take shortcuts such as driving to nearby errands (instead of walking).

## TORCHED CALORIES

Just 10 minutes of moderate exercise dials up your metabolism for an hour or longer, reports the journal *Science Translational Medicine*. Researchers found that levels of molecules involved in calorie burning changed significantly an hour after a 10-minute treadmill test—in some cases doubling among the fittest.

## LOWER ANXIETY

Studies suggest that small doses of regular exercise—we're talking about 10 to 20 minutes at a time—can result in temporary mood improvement or anxiety reduction. Exercise raises levels of serotonin, a feel-good hormone, while reducing your heart rate, blood pressure, and stress hormone levels.

## STRONGER FUTURE

A little exercise goes a long way when it comes to protecting your bones and heart down the road. Research shows that just 10 minutes of high-impact exercise (like plyometrics) three times a week can boost women's bone strength—a critical factor in staving off osteoporosis later in life. And doing just 30 minutes of weight training a week is linked to a 23 percent decrease in heart disease risk, according to Harvard researchers.

> *"The pessimist sees difficulty in every opportunity. The optimist sees opportunity in every difficulty."*
>
> —WINSTON CHURCHILL

# The Easiest Weight-Loss Secret Ever

▶ Here's the thing: Not all shortcuts are created equal. Most people who try to beat the laws of weight loss end up shooting themselves in the foot. Many women merely view weight loss as a means to an end. They set their sights on a quick fix, which typically translates into a month of early-morning spin classes and salads sans dressing. The problem? Almost anyone can suffer through a brutal month of overtraining and calorie restriction, but research has continually proven that people can't keep it up for long periods of time. It's simply not sustainable—physically or mentally. Cue a single roadblock—like a week off from the gym or that pint of Ben & Jerry's you swore you wouldn't polish off—and all of a sudden the wheels come off. When women set out on an all-or-nothing approach, they see one slipup as complete failure and they give up.

While small fluctuations on the scale are normal, this start-stop pattern usually leads to a significant increase or decrease of body weight (generally 10 pounds or more), and it's usually not a one-time deal. Experts refer to this as weight cycling—you know it as yo-yo dieting.

> *"Be not afraid of growing slowly,*
> *be afraid only of standing still."*
>
> —CHINESE PROVERB

According to a study published in the journal *American Psychologist*, dieters successfully lost up to 10 percent of their weight within the first 6 months on any number of diets; problem is, nearly two-thirds of dieters put the weight back on (sometimes gaining even more) within 5 years.

As if the roller-coaster scale wasn't tough enough, weight cycling can actually change your physiology, increasing a hunger hormone called ghrelin and decreasing a fullness hormone called leptin. The result: You feel hungrier and less satiated, and over time, the more diets you've been on, the harder it becomes to lose the weight. Researchers from Columbia University in New York City found that dieting can actually slow your resting metabolism and make it harder to maintain a stable weight post-diet. They reported that dieters may burn up to one-quarter fewer calories during exercise than those naturally at the same weight.

Just as yo-yo dieting hurts your waistline, having an on-again, off-again relationship with working out wreaks havoc on your health: People who gained 14 pounds in a month by exercising less and eating more were still up nearly 7 pounds from their original weight 30 months later, despite going back to their healthier patterns, according to a study in *Nutrition & Metabolism*. An irregular exercise pattern can raise your

## 🔒 SLIM-DOWN SECRET

Consistent exercisers who see working out as part of their lifestyle, rather than a way to change their appearance, have the most success keeping weight off.

body's natural set point (the weight your biological system naturally tries to maintain) and make it harder to dip below that number. And research shows that bouts of vigorous exercise followed by weeks of inactivity can increase fat levels and put excess strain on your cardio-vascular system.

But your relationship with healthy eating and exercise doesn't have to be so hot and cold. In fact, *ignoring* strict guidelines could be the secret to a successful slimdown. A study published in the *International Journal of Obesity* found that people with a flexible approach to eating—one that allows for sweets and other perceived slipups—had a better track record of maintaining weight loss than dieters with an all-or-nothing strategy. So if some days you're too busy for even a few minutes of exercise or you slip up from your diet, you can give yourself a break. Because here's the bigger picture: It's what you do most of the time—not all the time—that makes a difference. When overweight subjects in a study made several small lifestyle shifts—such as eating breakfast, having as many veggies as they'd like with each meal, and watching TV for only as long as they'd exercised that day—they dropped an average of 8 pounds in 2 weeks. And kept it off.

So when people say, "There are no shortcuts to any place worth going," here's what I think it really means: You can't skip the little things and jump ahead to the big finish. You have to put in the work every day. The road from dream to reality is laden with digestible and specific monthly, weekly, even daily challenges; bigger, long-term results are merely the sum of daily actions. But that doesn't mean the work has to be drastic or draining. Reaching milestones, however small, helps you stay focused and builds confidence. In fact, when you skip extreme regimens in favor of a handful of smaller strategies, the cumulative effect can be huge—and, more importantly, it won't feel as if you've given up your entire life to be fit.

# 5 RULES TO SMARTER WEIGHT LOSS

Goals are key—they're what keep you going when things start to suck. Use these five principles to make sure your goals are keeping you on the path to success.

### 1. Be Specific
Set out to just "tone up" and you're selling yourself short. Vague goals give people too much leeway and can lower their motivation to push themselves. So be precise and say, for example, that you want to lower your body fat by 10 percent or be able to run a 10-K.

### 2. Make It Measurable
You should be able to gauge and quantify your progress, both in the short and long term. Set micro (weekly) and macro (monthly) goals to keep yourself on track.

### 3. Stay within Reach
If you can barely find 20 free minutes in your day, don't set yourself up for failure by saying you'll run for 50 minutes 3 days a week.

### 4. Accept Reality
Even with the smartest plan and the strongest determination, your body can only handle so much. Sure, fast weight loss is possible, but if you drop more than about a pound and a half a week, you're most likely looking at muscle and water loss—not fat loss.

### 5. Time It Right
Deadlines help maintain a sense of significance and keep your goals a priority. Give yourself a year to drop 75 to 100 pounds, 4 to 6 months to train for a marathon (if you're a new runner), and 2 months to lose 10 to 12 percent of your body fat.

*"Nothing is impossible. The word itself says 'I'm possible.'"*

—AUDREY HEPBURN

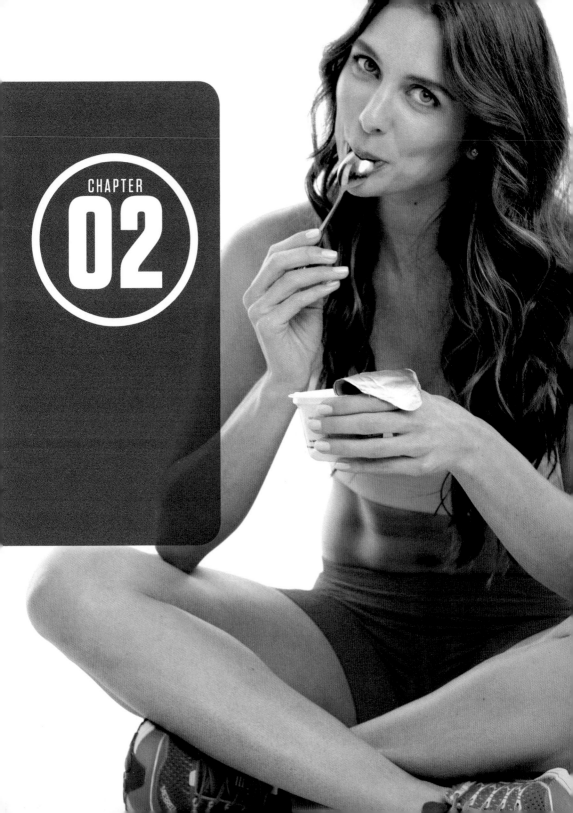

CHAPTER

02

# Upgrade Your Diet

*Painless tips for reinventing your relationship with food*

There's a reason you're reading this chapter before anything related to fitness and working out. In the battle against your waistline, you need to start where it matters most—and that means your daily food choices. All too often our routines look something like this: rush from the office (where you've been sitting most of the day) to the gym, sweat it out in spin class for an hour, and then pick up something to eat on the way home. Our nutrition needs have taken a backseat. But when your goal is fat loss, daily diet is one of the most—if not the single most—important pieces of the equation. Once that's on track, you can add effective (read: not excessive) exercise.

Unfortunately, healthy eating comes with a ton of perceived roadblocks: It's too expensive, too time consuming, too complicated, too strict, or too bland and boring. Maybe that's why it's also one area where people feel the most desperate.

# # BY THE NUMBERS

## 45

Percentage of people who eat fewer than five home-cooked dinners per week. And 17 percent don't even eat three.

They'll try anything that promises a solution to the number of potential pitfalls—and then they're devastated when it doesn't work.

For someone who is trying to lose weight for the first or 50th time, fad diets just won't work. Like I said earlier, when people do (or in this case, eat) things that are fast, easy, and enjoyable, they're more likely to repeat that choice. The more regular those habits become, the greater the scale will shift.

This isn't a diet program. It's a way to shift your mindset about eating so that you can completely transform your waistline—and your life. Smart nutrition is crucial, but as you'll see in the following pages, that doesn't mean it has to be complicated. Consider this: If you cut out just 96 calories from your daily diet, you'll be 10 pounds lighter 1 year from today—and that's *without* exercise or any strict diet programs.

# Bring It Home

▶ You may have heard the saying: "Abs are made in the kitchen." While that's true, there's some crucial fine print that's not often highlighted: It totally depends on who's cooking.

In 2009, Americans began spending more money eating out than preparing meals at home. In fact, total food dollars spent on out-of-home foods have increased 97 percent over the past 40 years. People aren't hitting up the drive-thru for their health: They do it because of the convenience. In fact, when researchers at the University of Minnesota School of Public Health surveyed adults about their attitudes toward fast foods, there was no link between frequency of fast-food intake and perceived healthful-

 **SHAPE-UP** SETBACK

People who regularly ate fast food over 6 years were 41 percent more likely to become depressed than those who avoided the greasy grub, reports the journal *Public Health Nutrition*. Scientists believe the high trans fats content may interfere with the brain's ability to produce certain mood-stabilizing neurotransmitters. For your physical and mental health, limit drive-thru trips and eat more fruits and vegetables.

Cook at home just 3 days a week and you could lose a pound a week. And the benefits go beyond the scale: People who cook often have a healthier relationship with food and are more likely to be satisfied by what they eat. In fact, researchers have found that women who take a forward-thinking approach to food and cooking (meaning they try new recipes, plan meals, and shop with a list) have a higher intake of vegetables.

ness of fast food; however, frequency of intake was significantly associated with perceived convenience and dislike toward cooking.

In short, they see it as a shortcut.

# THE COST OF EATING OUT

Check out how your meal changes depending on where it came from. Then consider the instant calorie savings you can score by cooking these foods at home.

**KEY:** RESTAURANT    HOME-COOKED

### PIZZA (per slice)

210 calories,
11 g total fat, 4 g saturated fat

187 calories,
5.5 g total fat, 2 g saturated fat

### GRILLED CHEESE

430 calories,
26.5 g total fat, 8 g saturated fat

270 calories,
15.5 g total fat, 9.5 g saturated fat

### STEAK

655 calories,
47.5 g total fat, 21 g saturated fat

243 calories,
8 g total fat, 2.5 g saturated fat

### PASTA

867 calories,
34 g total fat, 15 g saturated fat

422 calories,
10.5 g total fat, 2.5 g saturated fat

### PIE (per slice)

533 calories,
30 g total fat, 11 g saturated fat

355 calories,
17 g total fat, 5 g saturated fat

### ENCHILADA

1,315 calories,
65 g total fat, 25 g saturated fat

304 calories,
10 g total fat, 3 g saturated fat

I've been there. After a hectic day, when I know I don't have anything prepped or planned at home, it feels infinitely

easier to order takeout. But here's the thing: For the points it scores in convenience, eating out deducts them tenfold in calorie control. Experts estimate that eating at a restaurant increases your total calorie intake by 36 percent compared to eating at home. What's worse, you probably don't have a clue how many calories your entrée really contains: According to recent data from the University of Arkansas, the average diner underestimates each meal by up to 600 calories. Still need more reasons to eat in? Ninety-six percent of entrées sold in American chain restaurants contain more than one-third of the USDA's daily recommendations for calories, sodium, and total fat or saturated fat.

# Get Out of the Gym— And Into the Kitchen!

▶ One of the best pieces of fitness advice I received early in my job at *Women's Health* was: "You can't out-exercise a bad diet." If there's one thing you pick up from this chapter, it should be that. Why? Even top trainers will tell you that when it comes to losing body fat, it doesn't matter how often, how hard, or how long you work out—nutrition is going to be the key to your success. Building muscle is crucial for increased definition and boosting your metabolism, but if you want to get serious about getting in shape, you've got to realign your priorities. It's all about the food.

## Eating Right Outweighs Exercise

Starting an exercise program for the sole purpose of burning fat or losing weight is counterproductive. Researchers at the University of Minnesota pitted calorie restriction without exercise against cardio workouts with no dietary changes. The diet-only women lost significantly more weight in 8 weeks than those who exercised. (Don't cancel your gym membership just yet: The same study found that women lost the most weight when they combined diet and exercise.)

## Your Workout May Not Be Working

Or at least not as well as you think it is. People grossly overestimate how many calories they burn during exercise, especially when they think it's high intensity. It doesn't help when your boot-camp instructor says each class blasts 1,000 calories (a total exaggeration) or you check the counters on cardio machines (ellipticals have been reported to overestimate expenditure by 42 percent).

Estimating calorie output can be an inexact science; it involves factors like age, weight, body temperature, metabolic rate, and hormonal changes (to name a few) that are complicated, difficult to track, and ever-fluctuating. A bigger problem: Women sometimes use these assumptions about their workout to make decisions on how they eat for the rest of the day. Translation: When you believe your workout just torched 800 calories, you feel less guilty about the whip on your Frap-

 **2-SECOND LIFE CHANGER**

To help combat the inaccurate calorie-burn counts on some cardio machines, increase your calorie-burn goal by 30 percent. So if you go to the gym with the intention of burning 300 calories, aim for 390 instead.

puccino or those cookies after dinner. Focus on the muscle-building, metabolism-revving perks of your workout, rather than making your calorie-burn total the primary goal.

## Your Workout Can Work Against You

Moderately active women typically need about 1,800 to 2,200 calories a day to maintain their weight. To drop pounds, you'll need to shave anywhere from 250 to 500 calories a day from that total. Seems simple, right? Not quite. According to a study published in the *Journal of Sports Medicine and Physical Fitness*, college students consumed up to three times more calories than they burned during their last workout. Researchers believe that following exercise people may be less mindful of what they're putting into their mouths. Not only that, many women also tend to be less active throughout the rest of the day (by, say, not taking the stairs or spending more downtime on the couch): Research-ers at the University of South Carolina found that women burned 70 fewer calories during the day after doing a hard workout compared with days they didn't hit the gym.

## Exercise Can Happen Anytime, Anywhere

Think of all the opportunities you have to be active in between work-outs—taking the stairs instead of the elevator, walking across the office instead of sending an e-mail, or riding a bike instead of taking a cab. These on-the-go activities help you sneak in exercise without really even thinking about it.

Mindless, on-the-move eating? Yeah, usually doesn't help your weight-loss efforts. This is because mobile foods, although convenient, tend to be the ones most laden with fat, sugar, and sodium. Snacks in general have more calories than ever before.

# HUNGER GAMES

How you feel after working out—exhausted, drained, and possibly ravenous—can reinforce the idea that you burned a ton of calories and your body needs more fuel. (Not to mention, make you believe you deserve a treat.) While serious athletes need extra calories to offset their demanding training, the average woman has enough glycogen stored in her muscles and liver to power her through a workout.

That said, a 200-calorie snack (a mix of carbs and protein) during the hour after your workout can help muscle recovery efforts and restore glycogen supplies so you won't reach for candy later. Just remember to figure these calories into your daily count.

# Supermarket Survival Guide

▶ The first step to cooking up tasty, fat-shedding meals at home is putting the right stuff in your cart. It's easy to get tripped up by endless varieties, deceptive packaging, and the idea that shopping for healthy food means shelling out extra cash. These healthy-eating tips will save you time, money—and calories—before you hit the checkout line.

## SHOP IN YOUR UNDERWEAR

Web sites such as Amazon.com have gotten into the grocery business. They offer the same popular brands, and their prices rival Sam's Club and other bulk-buy places, so you'll save on gas as well as food. What's more, the shipping is usually free once your order hits $25.

## DON'T BE A BASKET CASE

Dashing into the store to pick up a few things? Don't grab a basket. If you're limited to what you can carry, you're more likely to avoid impulse purchases.

## FLY SOLO

Your guy may insist on pricey filet mignon instead of the pork loin that's on sale; your kids may bug you to buy a box of sugary and expensive cereal. Go shopping on your own and you'll be more likely to stick to the list you wrote before you left.

## DON'T SKIP THE FREEZER AISLE

Many people think if it's not fresh, it's not good. Good news: Because frozen and canned produce are flash-frozen or processed right at harvest

# # BY THE NUMBERS

## 32

Percentage drop in impulse buys when you use the self-checkout line.

time, they may be more nutritious than fresh produce that's been shipped all over the globe. Not to mention they're more affordable, and because they don't spoil as quickly, you're less likely to throw your money in the trash. So while fresh, local produce is ideal when it's in season, don't turn up your nose at frozen or canned goods. Having produce at home, even if it's in the freezer or a cabinet, means you're more likely to include more fruits and veggies in your daily diet.

## EAT BREAKFAST—ALL DAY LONG

Your go-to a.m. foods—eggs, fruit, cereal, oatmeal—tend to be both the most nutritious and inexpensive foods you eat all day, and they fill you up so you won't binge later. In fact, one of the easiest ways to cut down on costs while boosting your nutrition is to eat breakfast foods for lunch and dinner occasionally.

## SHOP WITH THE SLIM WOMEN

You know all those ingredients you can't pronounce when you read the labels of some packaged foods? Many are chemical additives that not only foil the spoilage process, but can also mess with your body's natural taste and appetite regulators. The solution? Aim to make the majority of your list single-ingredient products. This means you'll spend more time in the outer edges of the store—in the produce, meat, and dairy sections, where researchers have found that thinner women frequently shop.

## SAVVY SWAPS

Sure there are certain tastes that pair oh so perfectly together—buffalo wings and blue cheese, or peaches and your mom's cobbler. This doesn't mean there are no acceptable substitutions. Blue cheese pricey at the market? Try feta cheese or goat cheese. Apricots or nectarines on sale? Ditch your plan to pick up peaches and use those instead. Price for pine nuts too high for your budget? Almonds, pecans, or walnuts work just as well. The point is, you can always adapt—and you might even strike a new beloved flavor combination.

## LOOK HIGH AND LOW

Food manufacturers pay premium prices to ensure that their products sit on the middle shelf where our eyes naturally fall as we walk down each aisle, and that fee is undoubtedly passed on to shoppers. When you hit up the soup, pasta, and packaged-goods aisles, you'll find better deals—and generally healthier food—by shopping most heavily from the top and bottom shelves.

## KNOW YOUR ORGANICS

Organics cost more, so save money when you can. A report from the Environmental Working Group shows that fruits with thick skins like bananas, avocados, and oranges are generally safe in conventional form, while produce with edible or no skin—think celery, peaches, strawberries, and apples—is more likely to carry pesticides or chemical fertilizers.

# Cooking Rules That Will Change Your Life

▶ You don't have to be a Top Chef to create tasty, quick, and healthy meals at home. Use the following guidelines to make cooking and eating at home easier, faster, and more enjoyable—all without compromising your weight-loss efforts.

## BE FLEXIBLE

Ingredients aren't set in stone. If you have a bag of unused mushrooms in the fridge but the recipe calls for eggplant, chances are the 'shrooms will do just fine. Don't want to spend $3 on a bunch of celery just to use a single stalk? Omit it. You like pork chops more than chicken breast? Switch it. The point is, if you understand the basic techniques (which you'll learn on page 34) and have an idea of what tastes good together, the possibilities for creation in the kitchen are infinite.

## SEASON TO YOUR TASTE

When you see salt, pepper, or other spices listed in a recipe, keep this in mind: Your mouth is more accurate than a measuring spoon. Taste and adjust as early and often as possible. And, just like your ingredient list, seasonings can be swapped, dropped, added, or tweaked based on what you like, what you have, and how it's tasting.

## TREAT YOURSELF

Not just when it comes to calories (which, of course, is important to do from time to time), but also with the quality of food you buy. Americans spend less of their income on food than any other country in the world, yet our waistlines are growing quicker than any other population's. Adding a few dollars to your food budget in order to secure omega-3-rich grass-fed beef or glistening wild Alaskan salmon fillets is money well spent. If it's something that will help you look, feel, and function better—not to mention enjoy your meal more—it's worth the extra few bucks.

## LEARN TO LOVE LEFTOVERS

"Not that again!" While day-after meals tend to get a bad rap, many foods can actually taste better the next day. But reheat leftovers using the wrong method and you'll sacrifice moisture, texture, and any shot at having a satisfying second helping. Follow these three rules to breathe delicious life back into last night's healthy dinner.

**MAKE IT FAST.** You might think that since leftovers are already cooked, slow reheating would be ideal because it would prevent over-zapping them. In reality, slow reheating allows food to stay in the "danger zone"—between 40° and 140°F—for too long. Best to blast food with high heat—325°F at the very lowest—for a short time to take it from cool to hot quickly.

**STOCK IT.** Safety aside, taste and texture are hugely important factors to consider when reheating leftovers. And sadly, the reheating process too often leaves foods dry and unpalatable. Your new secret weapon: reduced-sodium chicken stock. Splash a bit on top of whatever you're reheating—pastas, meats, even vegetables—and the moisture will be reabsorbed by the food, bringing life and flavor back to the dish.

**DRESS IT UP.** As often as possible, add a layer of fresh flavor to leftovers after they've been heated. Pasta and soups benefit from a sprinkle of fresh parsley or basil, plus a drizzle of olive oil. Stir-fries could use some chopped scallion, toasted peanuts, and a spritz of lime. Meat and fish scream out for some fresh lemon juice and a sprinkling of flaky sea salt.

## HAVE THE RIGHT TOOLS

Here are the essentials you need to build a basic kitchen—and the extras you can invest in once you get started.

*START WITH . . .*

Cast-iron skillet

Grater

Knives (chef knife and paring
   knife)

Measuring cups and spoons

Medium saucepan

Mixing bowls

Muffin pans

Nonstick skillets

Rubber cutting board

Utensils: tongs, rubber spatula,

Y-shaped peeler

Wire mesh colanders

*THEN GET . . .*

Blender

Salad spinner

Serrated knife

Slow cooker

Wooden spoon

## *"The best way to predict the future is to create it."*

—ABRAHAM LINCOLN

# PANTRY POWERHOUSES

## Here are three body-slimming essentials.

### Canned Whole Peeled Tomatoes

Here's a secret: Most great Italian restaurants' red sauce is made with canned tomatoes. They're picked at the height of tomato season and canned instantly, preserving the intensely sweet, acidic flavor of summer tomatoes.

**Use It:** Combine with olive oil and salt for a perfect pizza sauce; use as the base for a slow-cooked dish, like baked chicken breasts; make delicious pasta sauce by simmering with onions, garlic, and red-pepper flakes.

### Chicken Stock

Restaurants use butter and cream as the base for sauces, which explains the high calorie totals. Using chicken (or vegetable or beef) stock—to moisten stuffing, build sauces, braise meat and vegetables— gives you flavor with minimal caloric impact.

**Use It:** Combine with equal parts red or white wine, plus shallots and herbs, and boil until reduced to sauce consistency (use on steak or chicken); stretch a pasta sauce by adding a few splashes of stock; add a few cups to a roasting pan you cooked meat in with a few pinches of flour and a pat of butter for instant gravy.

### Balsamic Vinegar

Perfect for building salad dressings and marinades, caramelizing onions, braising meat in a slow cooker, or pickling veggies.

**Use It:** Combine with equal parts soy sauce, plus chopped garlic, for a great steak or chicken marinade; mix with 2 parts olive oil, a small spoonful of Dijon mustard, and salt and pepper for an all-purpose vinaigrette; cover onions or cucumbers with balsamic for 10 minutes for an instant pickle; toss with chopped strawberries and pour over vanilla ice cream.

# SLIM DOWN YOUR PANTRY

Stock your kitchen with these ingredients and delicious, fat-torching meals will always be just minutes away.

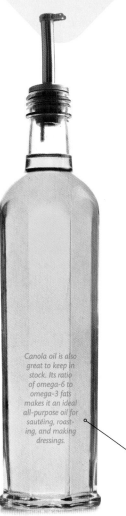

Canola oil is also great to keep in stock. Its ratio of omega-6 to omega-3 fats makes it an ideal all-purpose oil for sautéing, roasting, and making dressings.

**Almonds**

**Applesauce**
Use it instead of oil in your baked goods.

Perfect topper for oatmeal and salads.

**Barbecue sauce**
Look out for bottles with high sugar.

**Canned beans**
Try black, cannellini, pinto, chickpeas, or lentils.

People who eat ⅔ cup of beans per day have lower blood pressure and smaller waist sizes compared to those who don't eat beans.

**Canned tuna, chicken, crabmeat**

**Chili powder**

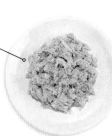

**Chili sauce**
It makes everything taste better.

**Curry powder**
This blend of turmeric, cinnamon, and coriander has disease-fighting properties.

Conventional albacore tuna contains about three times as much mercury as light tuna.

**Dried oregano**
Just as good dried as fresh.

**Dried rosemary**
It will keep for 6 months (to test, rub the leaves with your fingers—it should smell potent).

**Dried thyme**
If substituting for fresh, use ⅓ less than recipe calls for.

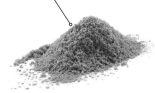

**Extra-virgin olive oil**

Punch up everything from your eggs to your tuna salad.

## Fruit spread

*Choose one made with 100% fruit and with no added sugar or high-fructose corn syrup.*

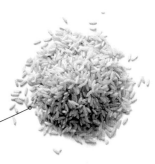

## Garlic powder

*Sub ⅛ teaspoon in place of one clove of garlic.*

## Ground cinnamon

*Sprinkle on oatmeal, over broiled grapefruit, or in a latte.*

## Ground cumin

*This spice can combat stress and amp up your memory.*

*Skip reduced fat—they swap healthy fats for fillers like sugar.*

## Panko bread crumbs

*Get the crunchy texture of your favorite fried foods for a fraction of the calories.*

## Paprika

*Sprinkle on fish or chicken.*

## Peanut butter (or almond butter)

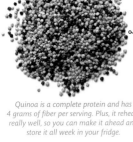

## Quinoa, brown rice, whole wheat couscous

*Prepare them ahead of time and store for fast weekly meals.*

*Quinoa is a complete protein and has 4 grams of fiber per serving. Plus, it reheats really well, so you can make it ahead and store it all week in your fridge.*

## Red or white wine vinegar

*Use as a base for salad dressings or marinades.*

## Red-pepper flakes

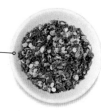

## Reduced-sodium soy sauce

*Not just for sushi—add to salad dressings and marinades, too.*

*Make an instant zesty red sauce by adding to canned tomatoes.*

## Salsa

*Top it on practically anything—seriously.*

## Sugar-free syrup

*Use it to sweeten yogurt—and even marinades.*

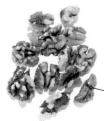

## Walnuts

*To bring out their flavor, toast them for 10 minutes then chop and add to salads.*

*Studies conducted by the National Institutes of Health found that the omega-3 fatty acids in walnuts keep the stress hormones cortisol and adrenaline in check.*

## Whole wheat flour

*Use about ¾ cup for every 1 cup of all-purpose flour in recipes.*

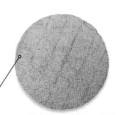

*Wrap up a breakfast scramble or chicken fajita—or use as a personal-size pizza crust.*

## Whole wheat tortillas

# Kick Your Kitchen Skills Up a Notch

➤ Cutting back on takeout doesn't mean you have to eat a bowl of cereal for dinner every night. Despite what you see in foodie magazines and on TV these days, all you need to prepare delicious, calorie-conscious meals at home are a few simple and straightforward cooking techniques.

## ROASTING

Roasting caramelizes the sugars in meats and vegetables, developing their natural sweetness, so it's a great way to enhance flavor without adding calories. And because the oven does almost all the work, very little prep is required.

**BEST FOR:** Whole chicken, beef or pork roast, and fatty fish like salmon. Also, thicker root vegetables like potatoes, sweet potatoes, Brussels sprouts, carrots, parsnips, and squash; that's not to say asparagus, peppers, zucchini, and tomatoes can't be roasted—just keep an eye on them, since they can burn easily.

**HOW TO DO IT:** Preheat the oven to 400°F. Lightly coat the ingredients with olive oil and season with salt, pepper, and your favorite dried herbs. Use the digital thermometer to determine when meats are done. Vegetables are ready when they start to brown on the outside and are tender on the inside, usually about 35 to 40 minutes (give them a quick toss after about 20 minutes).

## BROILING

By putting food directly under exposed high heat, broiling gives food a crispy texture yet keeps it moist and juicy inside—all without adding much oil or fat.

# (DON'T!) JUST HEAT IT

## Though convenient, the microwave reheats

food unevenly and has an uncanny ability to make crisp foods soggy and moist foods dry. Take the time to reheat your food correctly and you'll be rewarded.

### Pizza

No more soggy slices.Place one or two slices in a cast-iron skillet set over low heat. Warm until the bottoms have crisped up slightly and the cheese has remelted. (For more slices or a large pie, heat on a baking sheet in a preheated 500°F oven for 4 to 5 minutes.)

### Steak, roasted chicken, and pork chops

Leave the meat out on the counter for 20 minutes before cooking. Heat a thin film of oil in a cast-iron skillet over medium heat, then add the meat and cook for 2 to 3 minutes, or until there's a nice crust on one side. Flip and place the whole skillet into a preheated 350°F oven for 5 to 7 minutes, depending on the thickness.

### Chili, soup, and braises

The meat and vegetables in these dishes absorb liquid as the leftovers sit, so to achieve proper consistency, heat in a large saucepan with up to a cup of reduced-sodium chicken or vegetable stock (or water), and stir constantly to ensure even heating.

### Pasta and Asian noodle dishes

Noodles soak up moisture as they lie with sauces and oils, so it's a good idea to separate them whenever possible. Add the pasta to a heated nonstick skillet with ¼ cup of reduced-sodium chicken stock or water per serving. Cook until the noodles are hot and the sauce is bubbling, about 3 to 4 minutes. Garnish with fresh chopped herbs (basil or parsley) and grated cheese.

### Burgers and chicken sandwiches

Preheat the oven to 350°F. Put the meat on a baking sheet and place in the oven for 5 to 6 minutes, until the outside is hot to the touch. Toast a fresh bun and apply new produce and condiments.

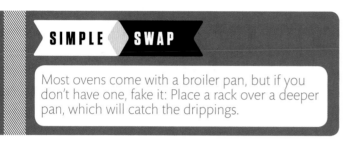

SIMPLE SWAP

Most ovens come with a broiler pan, but if you don't have one, fake it: Place a rack over a deeper pan, which will catch the drippings.

**BEST FOR**: Thin cuts of meat or fish that will cook quickly and taste great with a golden-brown exterior. Think flank or skirt steaks, lamb or pork chops, and all kinds of fish.

**HOW TO DO IT**: All the meat needs is a dash of salt and freshly ground pepper; drizzle fish with olive oil and lemon juice. Set the broiler to high; if your oven doesn't have a built-in broiler, adjust your top oven rack so that it is about 8 inches from the top heating element. The thickness of the cut and how well done you like your meat will determine how long to leave it in—ranging from 3 minutes per side for a thin rare steak to 9 minutes per side for a thick well-done one.

## BOILING

It's a fast (not to mention, damn easy) way to cook food, and since you're using only water, you're not adding fat or calories. But while it seems foolproof, many people make a few common mistakes when boiling. Use these tips to do it better.

**1:** Pasta or vegetables such as broccoli and spinach do best on high heat in a quick, rolling boil. Soups, sauces, and hearty vegetables such as potatoes and carrots yield the most flavor and tenderness with a slow simmer.

**2:** To cook chicken, cover with water and add veggies or herbs; cover the pot and bring to a boil, then lower to a simmer for 90 minutes.

**3:** Don't bother putting oil in pasta water—it doesn't prevent sticking. Instead, toss pasta with a tablespoon of olive oil after you've drained it.

## SAUTÉING

This quick-cooking technique involves constantly tossing or stirring the food with a tablespoon or two of oil or butter over high heat. It preserves the natural flavor, texture, and color of foods.

**BEST FOR:** Naturally tender cuts, such as beef tenderloin, fish fillets, or chicken breast (tougher cuts require too much cooking time) and quick-cooking vegetables, such as asparagus, peppers, broccoli, onions, sugar snap peas, and mushrooms.

**HOW TO DO IT:** Add just enough oil to coat the skillet, then heat over medium-high heat for a minute or two before tossing in your ingredients. Before adding all the ingredients, test the heat level with a single piece; it should sizzle when it hits the skillet. (If you add the food too early, it will release its liquid and your dish will turn out soggy.) Cook, tossing frequently; for how long depends on what you're making. If you're cooking a mix of foods, brown your meat first, then add aromatics (garlic, onions) and vegetables.

 **2-SECOND LIFE CHANGER**

Especially when sautéing vegetables, seasoning at the right time is crucial. Salt early and vegetables give off liquid and create steam for a soft cook. If you're looking for caramelization, salt at the last second.

**Quick Tip:** *When chopping ingredients for a sauté, cut everything into uniform pieces so your food cooks evenly, at the same rate.*

## BRAISING

It's the most time consuming of the group, but cooking food (usually meat) in a flavorful liquid over low heat for several hours yields succulent, melt-in-your-mouth meals that absolutely scream with flavor. It may not be your go-to option during the week, but it's a great choice for cooking large portions of meat ahead of time to have in your fridge for leftovers.

**BEST FOR**: Dark-meat chicken still on the bone (legs and thighs), pork shoulders, or beef chuck roasts (pot roasts). Slow-cooking the meat in liquid until the fat breaks down is what makes it so tender. Adding vegetables rounds out the flavor, but since they'll be cooking for long periods of time in liquid, choose ones like carrots and potatoes.

**HOW TO DO IT**: Brown the meat in a pot on the stove top, then add your vegetables and pour in enough liquid to reach one-half to two-thirds of the way up the meat; cover. Almost any liquid will do, but the easiest to use is stock. Match a reduced-sodium version with your main ingredient (beef stock for beef, and so on); when in doubt, use chicken stock. Herbs and spices will infuse the meal with flavor when added to the braising liquid, and you can also add in other liquids, such as beer or wine. Simmer over low heat or in the oven at a low temperature, keeping the pot covered. You don't have to turn the meat, though if you want, you can do so halfway through. Cook beef and other meats for 60 to 90 minutes per pound; for a whole chicken, count on 45 minutes per pound.

Quick Tip: *Keep portions to no more than 3 ounces per serving—the best meats for braising are full of fat.*

## SWEATING

Use this method to cook vegetables without adding fat. Heat a saucepan or skillet over very low heat (if you must use oil, make it less than 1 tablespoon). Add your veggie—chopped onions are typical, but you can use whatever the recipe calls for—and salt, and stir. The idea is to avoid browning the onions and instead force them to release their juices. Once they do (within about 10 minutes), cook another 5 minutes before adding other ingredients.

## POUNDING PROTEIN

You may see recipes that call for pounding a piece of meat, especially chicken, into a thinner cutlet. The reason is that meat with a uniform

# PREP KITCHEN

## Cut down on the time it takes to get veggies ready to cook with these super-simple tips.

### Butternut squash

Cut off the top and very bottom so the squash will sit on a flat surface without wobbling. Stand it on one end and halve it lengthwise, then peel off the outer rind.

### Tomato

Cut a small *X* into the skin. Drop the tomato into boiling water and wait 15 seconds; fish it out with a slotted spoon and then drop it into ice water. The skin will slide right off.

### Corn on the cob

Nuke two unhusked ears on high power for 6 to 8 minutes. Then cut off the bottom half-inch and slip the cob from the husk. The kernels will be tender and, even better, silk free.

### Eggplant

Salt slices and let sit for 20 minutes, then squeeze and pat dry. Salt draws out the bitter juice and keeps the spongy flesh from absorbing too much oil during cooking.

### Onion

To avoid crying, freeze the onion for 10 minutes. Doing so prevents the release of the enzymes that irritate your eyes.

thickness cooks quicker and more evenly. The process is super simple, too: Take out a large cutting board and lay the protein on top. Cover with a few layers of plastic wrap and use a meat mallet (or a heavy-bottomed pan) to hit the meat.

## BREADING CHICKEN

For moist, crunchy chicken, you need full bread-crumb coverage. This method works for nearly all pan- and oven-fried recipes.

> **STEP 1:** Cover and pound the chicken until ¼ inch thick.
> **STEP 2:** Coat in flour, then dip in beaten egg.
> **STEP 3:** Fully cover the chicken with panko bread crumbs.

# 10 Secrets of the Slim

➥ Launch into pretty much any diet plan and you're bound to lose some weight. It's not magic; suddenly, you're not randomly grazing—you're following a meal plan and eating with a purpose, even if that purpose is based on pseudoscience or radical theories. The problem is, your brain is a calorie hog, and it takes an immense amount of concentration to stick to a complicated diet. Not to mention, from day one, most don't feel sustainable—so you know from the get-go it's a temporary fix. The super-simple principles you'll find throughout this chapter make losing weight doable, not daunting. They may even feel too easy or basic to work, but that's the point. Their shortcuts may not be as obvious and their results may not show up as quickly as fad diets'. But while not as quick, they're lasting. By trading in your old dieting ways, you'll save time in the long run because you'll be able to sustain these, and therefore maintain your lighter weight. Learn to eat healthy, one meal at a time, by ditching deprivation and shifting to a new way of eating—and say goodbye to your fickle and fluctuating relationship with the scale.

# 1. Take Baby Steps to Better

Let's be realistic: You aren't going to trade in potato chips for kale chips, fried chicken for broiled, or ice cream for frozen grapes overnight. And that's why most diets fail you. They often deprive you of foods that your body is accustomed to, and replace them with uberhealthy choices that sound the alarm to let your brain know you're on a diet—a move that sets you up for out-of-control cravings and, eventually, weight-gain relapse.

Instead of going cold turkey, transition from less healthy eats to better ones in baby steps. For the first week, don't even make it about the food, just focus on drinking six to eight glasses of water a day. Then, during the second week, trade ½ cup of your rice or pasta at dinner for the same amount of vegetables. Then, try ordering your bacon cheeseburger on a bed of lettuce rather than a bun, and so on. These small moves will build confidence and teach your body to enjoy healthy foods that satisfy hunger—without any frustration or burnout. Success, then, results from targeted efficiency rather than probability.

The chart on the next pages demonstrates how to wean yourself off less-than-ideal grub. Spend 2 to 4 weeks at each stage—the reward system in your brain needs time to adapt. I promise, after a few weeks you won't be focusing on the changes to your plate, only the ones to your waistline.

# BREAKFAST

| BAD | GOOD | BETTER | BEST |
|---|---|---|---|
| **Store-Bought Packaged Muffins** | **Homemade Blueberry-Yogurt Muffins** | **Two Scrambled Eggs, One Package of Plain Instant Oatmeal** | **Omelet Wrap** |
| Oh, don't they look tasty! Too bad most are made with white flour and an overload of sugar—a 3-incher has about 550 calories. | Using wheat germ gives these muffins a shot of fiber and protein, plus they have only 120 to 130 calories each and keep the sugar and fat in check. (Find the recipe on page 271.) | Eggs are a complete protein, and having them in the morning can kick-start your metabolism. Pairing with oatmeal's healthy carbs will hold off hunger until lunch. | Use one egg and one egg white to save about 40 calories (compared with two whole eggs), veggies for low-cal fiber, 1 tablespoon of cheese, and a whole wheat wrap. Quick, filling, and delicious—a weight-loss trifecta. |

# SALAD

| BAD | GOOD | BETTER | BEST |
|---|---|---|---|
| **Iceberg Lettuce with 2 Tablespoons of Creamy Dressing** | **Romaine with 1 Tablespoon of Creamy Dressing** | **Romaine with 1 Tablespoon of Balsamic Vinaigrette** | **Baby Spinach with 1 Tablespoon of Balsamic Vinaigrette** |
| *Iceberg* doesn't exactly sound packed with sustenance, does it? You won't find the immune-boosting, disease-fighting powers that other greens boast, and the dressing adds about 15 grams of fat. | Romaine packs more antioxidants in its leaves, and cutting the dressing in half slashes an easy 70 calories. | Don't reach for the fat-free kind: The olive oil in the regular variety contains healthy fats to keep you satisfied longer. | Spinach leaves are full of B vitamins, which may help lower your risk for certain cancers. (Find even more super salads on page 277.) |

# CHIPS

| BAD | GOOD | BETTER | BEST |
|---|---|---|---|
| **Regular Potato Chips** | **Baked Potato Chips** | **Bean Chips** | **Kale Chips** |
| Frying anything adds fat and produces acrylamide, a chemical that's been identified as a possible carcinogen. | It's a step in the right direction, with 40 fewer calories and 8 grams less fat per serving. But white spuds aren't exactly a weight-loss superfood. | Many kinds have more calories than baked chips, but they're also packed with about 4 grams of protein and 5 grams of fiber per serving, so they're more filling. | These babies pack fiber, vitamin A, calcium for bone strength, vitamin C to grow cells, and vitamin K, which may help bone growth. They're simple to make at home, too (find a few recipes on page 321). |

# CHICKEN

| BAD | GOOD | BETTER | BEST |
|---|---|---|---|
| **Fried Chicken** | **Baked Chicken with Barbecue Sauce** | **Chicken Parmesan** | **Grilled or Baked Herb-Crusted Chicken** |
| That deliciously crunchy coating comes at a cost—usually anywhere up to 9 grams of saturated fat per serving. | You ditch the dangerous saturated fat, but most finger-licking sauces are loaded with sugar and salt. | Little or no sugar here, but keep the shredded cheese to 4 teaspoons max to control the fat and calories. | Compared to its fried counterpart, where you started, this flavor-packed alternative can save you nearly 7 grams of saturated fat and 200 calories. (Find 50 ways to cook better chicken on page 305.) |

# 2. Keep It Consistent

Make sure your approach to eating is one you can stick with. No crash diets or fads—which are literally defined by their fleeting status. Ask yourself, "Can I see myself eating like this forever?" If the answer is no, you need to change your approach. You should think of this as a permanent lifestyle shift.

And consistency doesn't just mean Monday through Friday either. Researchers have found that people who eat consistently day to day are one and a half times more likely to maintain their weight loss than those who diet only on weekdays. For most people, weekends mean relaxing their diet or indulging in a few splurges, and a study in the *Journal of Public Policy & Marketing* found that adults scarf down, on average, 419 extra calories each weekend.

At the same time, it's important to remember that one meal doesn't define your diet—and it doesn't mean you've failed or fallen off the wagon. So maybe you couldn't stop yourself from polishing off the entire caramel sundae (that came after the spinach dip and chicken quesadillas), but that's no reason to give up entirely. Instead, think of it this way: Every meal is a chance to start over and do it right. Follow up a fall from nutritional grace with healthy choices the next five times you eat. This means you'll be eating right more than 80 percent of the time. It's what you eat the majority of the time that impacts your waistline.

# 3. Take Control

Don't rely on hope and prayers to get the body you want. Investing just an hour or two on the weekend to get a jump start on preparing your meals for the week (cutting veggies, making marinades) will save you time and pounds in the long run. Creating a "menu" each week—say, grilled chicken with roasted vegetables on Monday night, yogurt with fresh fruit and granola for Tuesday's breakfast, and so on—creates a confident path to success. A survey by the Centers for Disease Control and Prevention found that almost 40 percent of people who lost a significant amount of weight and kept it off planned their weekly meals. When you don't map out your meals, you're too tempted to grab whatever's nearby, which is often high-calorie junk.

If arranging every meal feels too rigid, map out a list of potential options for your meals and snacks based on the foods you have available, instead. This will give you the flexibility to choose based on your tastes at the time, but the hard part (thinking of something to make) will already be out of the way. According to Dutch researchers, thinking about snacks and meals can actually help you stay lean. The study

# PEER PRESSURE

You always hear that support can boost your weight-loss goals, but it turns out that friends can be as corrupting as a platter of nachos at happy hour. In fact, 53 percent of women said that others pressured them to eat foods that weren't on their diet. Here's how survey respondents' slim-down efforts were sabotaged.

### How Others Interfered

**40%** Cooked and served food not on my diet

**35%** Made jokes about my diet

**31%** Ordered food for me that's not on my diet

### Pressures to Break a Diet

**56%** Didn't want to insult someone

**51%** Wanted to eat like everyone else

**41%** Didn't want to call attention to my diet

found that when asked questions like "What will you do if you get hungry 2 hours before your next meal?" thinner participants were better able to give healthy responses like "eat a handful of nuts."

Planning ahead can also help prevent slipups. How many times have you actually driven to the store late at night to pick up a pint of ice cream? Now, compare that to how many times you've raided your fridge. You're more likely to give in to a craving when the object you desire is close at hand. Simple solution: Make sure it's not. Do your meal brainstorming before you head to the grocery store and make a list of the ingredients you need for the upcoming week; sticking to just what you have outlined can help you skip impulse items, and you'll get in and out of the store quicker.

## 4. Find Your Own Frequency

Around the turn of the millennium, research began to sing the benefits of eating more frequently (as opposed to sticking to three main meals). The "graze, don't gorge" philosophy is based on the idea that having frequent small meals keeps your blood sugar steady, your metabolism ramped up, and your appetite in check. A big part of the logic is that going too long between meals—or skipping them completely—may lead to overeating later. It could even explain why women who skipped meals lost about 8 pounds less than those who ate more consistently, according to a study in the *Journal of the Academy of Nutrition and Dietetics*.

Here's the thing: Other research shows a link between obesity and eating more than three times a day, most notably in women. After all, more frequent nosh-ing means more opportunities to overeat. Plus, having to constantly think about what you're going to eat can be stressful, especially for emotional eaters.

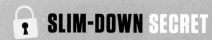

**SLIM-DOWN SECRET**

Planning ahead doesn't just apply to your at-home meals. When you're eating out, it's almost more crucial to have a plan; with so many tempting options, an impromptu order can easily wreck your diet. A surefire way to stay on track, no matter what restaurant you go to: Order a soup or salad as a starter and bypass the bread basket: Researchers found that people eat 47 percent more of a food when they start their meal with it.

The verdict: The mini-meal approach doesn't work for everyone—and it doesn't have to. You'll eat healthiest if you eat your way—meaning, if you prefer substantial meals fewer times a day, there's no reason to force yourself to do the opposite.

## 5. Eat Food You Actually Like

If eating nothing but raw foods, or locally sourced meat, or cabbage soup sounds enjoyable to you—go for it. But for the vast majority of people, these aren't maintainable eating options, they're diets. To be sustainable, you have to actually like, not just tolerate, the food you're being told to eat. If you don't, you start off knowing it's going to be a short-term gig, which could make you throw in the towel even sooner.

But while a strict program can be a great tool for resetting your eating habits, if it's not tailored to your schedule, budget, and personal preferences, it will eventually fail. That's not to say you won't see any results. In fact, any time you completely eliminate something from your diet—say, gluten, sugar, processed food, or booze—you tend to shed some weight. It's partly what bolsters the allure of fad diets—people "prove" they are effective by getting results.

## 2-SECOND LIFE CHANGER

There's a reason we're such suckers for holiday treats. Decades of research show that items we perceive as being in limited supply seem more desirable to us than nonscarce items. Give yourself a limited allotment of your favorite holiday treat (like a Starbucks Peppermint Mocha or McDonald's Shamrock Shake) and stick to it.

However, for a diet plan to work in the long run, it has to be meaningful to you. Does a particular diet call for a list of organic or fresh foods that cost more than your weekly take-home pay or might spoil before you can eat them? Find frozen varieties for a fraction of the cost that will keep if you're only cooking for one. Does your French-inspired meal plan call for blue cheese on everything, but you despise the taste? Switch to mozzarella, or Swiss, or feta cheese. Do you crave carbs every day, despite your resolve to stick to Atkins? The truth is, aside from medical or ethical reasons, there's no real payoff to nixing entire food groups. Instead of dropping carbohydrates, for example, refigure your approach to focus on making better choices on the sources (say, by swapping potatoes au gratin for a baked sweet potato or roasted fingerlings).

When it comes to weight loss, your total calorie intake is what matters the most. If you eat fewer calories than you burn on a cabbage-soup diet, you will lose weight. Likewise, if you eat more than you burn, the surplus can lead to weight gain, regardless of what foods those calories come from. By making meal decisions based on your tastes and preferences rather than on what your friend eats or the latest fad diet, you'll feel more satisfied by every meal.

# 6. Size Everything Up

While variables like meal timing and division of macronutrients are always hot topics to debate, there's one thing everyone should be able to agree on: Size matters.

Our portion-control meter doesn't register like it used to; in today's supersized society, our measure of a "just right" serving is far larger than it was just 30 years ago. This has impacted our ability to eye up proper portions. According to Purdue University researchers, the biggest problem with our snacking habits is that our

## SLIM-DOWN SECRET

People who learned skills for maintaining a steady weight before starting a diet were more likely to keep pounds off than those who dieted right away, according to a study in the *Journal of Consulting and Clinical Psychology*. Participants who mastered maintenance habits—like finding tasty low-cal swaps for high-cal foods and eating mindfully—regained only 3 pounds after a year, compared with 7 pounds among the diet-first group. Thinking things through when you're starting out harnesses your enthusiasm and channels it into keeping weight off—the part of dieting many people struggle with most, say the study authors.

between-meal bites have taken on actual meal-size proportions, and our actual meals have become feasts by comparison. It's not even because we're hungry: In one study, Pennsylvania State University researchers found that subjects ate 30 percent more food when presented with bigger portions, yet their perceived fullness didn't change.

Fad diets and nixed food groups have also contributed. Say you're following a sort of low-carb, high-protein diet, where 40 percent of your daily calories comes from protein, 40 percent from dietary fat, and 20 percent from carbohydrates. In this scenario, you can eat plenty of peanut butter or bacon (or peanut butter *and* bacon, a combination that creates one of my dad's favorite sandwiches) without gaining weight because of the overall calorie split. But when you veer off course or ditch the diet completely, you have to readjust those percentages. If you continue to eat the same portion sizes, but now with bread, you're likely getting more calories than you need, which can lead to weight gain.

There's another sneaky portion problem that you're likely not keeping a close eye on. Women often tell me (with great pride) about their healthy meal choices: They start their day with Greek yogurt with fresh berries and granola; snack on an apple with peanut butter or carrots and hummus; their lunchtime salad is topped with avocado, walnuts, hard-cooked eggs, and feta cheese; dinners are a well-balanced mix of brown rice, chicken, and roasted veggies. That all sounds fantastic, right? Of course, but there's a crucial question that needs to be asked, especially if these women are still struggling to hit their goal weight: "How much?" While the food choices are spot on, it is possible to have too much of a good thing. Downsize your dishes. People take less when they use smaller serving dishes and tall, narrow glasses instead of short wide ones, a study showed.

## 7. Track Feelings, Not Calories

Our tracking-app age has intensified this idea that a "calorie is a calorie"—that weight loss isn't really about what you eat, but how many calories you eat. As long as your weight-loss app says you came in under your daily caloric totals, it doesn't matter if you had two candy bars for lunch. While counting each and every

 **2-SECOND LIFE CHANGER**

Cornell University research shows that eating satisfaction is derived from the flavor intensity and visual impact of a meal, not necessarily the amount served. Kick your food up a notch with spices, which add flavor without the calories and fat.

# IN OR OUT?

**Think one of your favorite food** groups is on the health shame list? It may be time to bring it back to the table.

## Gluten

For those with a gluten intolerance, dropping the protein found in wheat, rye, and barley is necessary. If you try going sans gluten for a few weeks and notice no substantial difference, there's likely no need to drop it completely.

## Red Meat

Red meat may be higher in calories, fat, and saturated fat than, say, chicken or fish, but there are plenty of diet-friendly cuts—usually called round, tenderloin, or roast. Look for cuts labeled at least 95 percent lean, and keep your portion to 3 or 4 ounces—roughly the size of a smartphone.

## Dairy

Cutting back on the amount of dairy you eat can signal your body to make more fat cells, according to a study in the *American Journal of Clinical Nutrition*. When you don't have enough calcium in your body, it tries to hold on to what's there. This triggers the release of a compound called calcitriol, which increases the production of fat cells.

## Carbohydrates

People who make rice part of their daily diet weigh less than those who don't regularly eat the grain, according to a study in *Nutrition Today*. Besides being packed with belly-filling fiber and valuable nutrients, rice is also more likely to be paired with veggies and lean protein (think stir-fries and sushi) than fatty dishes such as pizza.

## Eggs

The incredible, edible egg is actually an excellent, affordable source of protein and B vitamins, and it may help you lose weight. A study in the *International Journal of Obesity* found that dieters who consumed two eggs for breakfast each day lost significantly more weight than those who consumed bagels.

calorie may help keep your intake in check, it can also take up way too much of your time and make you feel crazy.

For a minute, consider the irony of the whole eat-like-a-caveman approach to the Paleo Diet: Our prehistoric ancestors didn't diet. They didn't stress over contradicting rules like carbs versus no carbs, breakfast versus no breakfast. They didn't judge the food they were eating or worry about how many calories it contained. Their approach was much more intuitive: Find quality food (day-old meat or half-rotted vegetables wouldn't do), and eat enough to have energy to get through the tasks of the day.

## SIMPLE SWAP

*Pump up your protein intake.* Substituting meat, fish, dairy, and nuts for carbs can reduce the amount of fat around your middle. Researchers at McMaster University in Hamilton, Ontario, assessed the diets of 617 people and discovered that when they exchanged carbohydrates in favor of an equal amount of protein, they reduced overall belly fat.

If more of us adopted their mind-set rather than their menu, we might have better results—and, I'd argue, feel a lot less overwhelmed and bogged down by healthy eating. Researchers at the University of Texas at Austin found that women lost more weight by learning behavior-change strategies and minding their hunger cues than by fixating on external cues (like polishing off your plate) or diet rules (like eating a certain number of calories).

Try a little experiment: For 1 week, take a break from the numbers and, instead, keep track of when you eat and how you feel. Look for patterns. Do you always hit up your coworker's candy jar after a tough meeting? Do you graze before dinner out of boredom? Do you always crave ice cream after seeing a Dairy Queen commercial? Identifying and working to change these habits can help you slim down in the long run.

## 8. Lose the Labels

You thought I was talking about the ones on packaged foods, didn't you? That works, too, but it's not what I'm referring to. When it comes to nutrition, everyone today seems to be looking for a good guy and a bad guy. But putting a mental safety lock on "bad" foods doesn't guarantee results. According to a study in the *American Journal of Clinical Nutrition*, participants who restricted junk-food intake shed the same amount of weight as those who didn't. The researchers found that subjects who deprived themselves still splurged—just on other grub. It can also actually make you crave the off-limits food more: Women who suppressed thoughts about chocolate craved it more—and ate more when they gave in.

# SLIM-BODY EATS

Fat in any form packs more than twice the amount of calories as protein and carbs. A study published in the *New England Journal of Medicine* found that a diet high in healthy fats is superior to a low-fat diet, both in terms of weight loss and overall health benefits. Fat is filling and adds flavor to your meals—both of which help you avoid feeling deprived. But the source matters: Think nuts, salmon, avocados, and olive oil. Watch the portions: People often eat too much. Olive oil is the number one offender. A cup has close to 2,000 calories, and unless you're a stickler for measuring, it's easy to pour on more than the proper 2-teaspoon serving.

Even your positive association with healthy foods can expand your waistline: Turns out, the fewer calories you think a food has, the more of it you tend to eat. (In one study, people were shown a bowl of chili alone and another bowl next to a plate of greens—and they underestimated the number of calories in the chili with the salad.) Experts refer to it as the "health halo" effect, and manufacturers and restaurants use it against you by making foods sound healthier: A study in the *Journal of Consumer Research* found that people, particularly those with a history of dieting, tended to consume more when a food had a description like "fruit chews" than when the identical nosh was called "candy chews."

# 9. Snack Smarter

While they were instituted as small bites to keep hunger at bay between meals, today roughly one-quarter of the calories in the American diet come from snacks, according to a study published in the *Journal of Nutrition*.

And snack-size packaging, which supposedly was

introduced to help manage our portions, may only make matters worse. Researchers found that dieters inhaled significantly more calories from mini packs of cookies than from standard-size ones. When you finish one bag and still aren't satisfied (the portions are really small, after all), you dig into another—and then another.

Homemade servings are not likely to trigger the same overeating as store-bought packs, because the size of the food isn't deceptively smaller—the amount is limited, but to a portion that satisfies you. Reframe your definition of snacks from treats to a mini meal—like a packet of instant oatmeal with a few tablespoons of slivered almonds, instead of a candy bar.

## 10. Slow It Down

Dutch researchers found that big bites and fast chewing can lead to overeating. Participants who chewed larger bites of food for 3 seconds consumed 52 percent more food before feeling full than those who chewed small bites for 9 seconds. The reason: Tasting food for a longer period of time (no matter how much of it) signals your brain to make you feel full sooner. But it can take up to 10 minutes for your brain to get the message that your stomach is

 **2-SECOND LIFE CHANGER**

Make sure your appetite is real by picturing, say, a big steak or a gooey bowl of homemade macaroni and cheese. If it isn't appetizing, your "hunger" might just be boredom or thirst.

# MUNCH METER

## Some snacks can be downed with near abandon; others need to be reined in. See how some of your favorites measure up.

### All You Can Eat (Really!)
No need to limit these filling, low-cal treats.

- Air-popped popcorn
- Raw veggies such as jicama, sugar snap peas, and cherry tomatoes
- Steamed artichoke (dip in a warm mixture of fat-free plain Greek yogurt and Dijon mustard)
- Fresh berries
- Cucumber slices marinated in rice wine vinegar and topped with chopped red onions

### Take It Slow
Enjoy these healthy snacks; just don't go hog wild.

- One hard-cooked egg dusted with sea salt and black pepper (70 calories)
- A 1-ounce chunk of Parmesan (110 calories)
- Three slices of turkey breast wrapped in lettuce, with a little mustard (70 calories)

### Proceed with Caution
Portion control is key with these nutritious but high-cal eats.

- Half an avocado with lemon and sea salt (160 calories)
- ¼ cup of raisins or other dried fruit (123 calories)
- About 15 nuts or 1 tablespoon of all-natural nut butter (100 calories)
- 2 tablespoons of hummus (50 calories)

full. If you tend to inhale your food, you run the risk of stuffing yourself before realizing you're satiated.

The key to avoiding this button-popping feeling of regret is to eat before you're completely starving (like, say, a 6 on a hunger scale of 10) and spend 20 to 30 minutes on a meal. This is long enough to get that satiety signal, but not so long that you'll be tempted to go for a second helping. And be particularly mindful during dessert: Levels of certain chemicals rise when people eat their favorite foods, reports the *Journal of Clinical Endocrinology & Metabolism*, indicating that the food may turn on the brain's reward system, which overrides signals that you've had enough.

# Eat, Drink, and Still Shrink

▶ Dodge dieting pitfalls with these easy-to-execute tips.

## The Obstacle: Happy Hour

Between the drinks and the bar food, you could possibly put away 1,000 calories at happy hour. Alcohol stimulates your appetite and lowers your inhibitions, so you typically end up caving to cravings— or just eating whatever's around you. The fix: Decide how many drinks you'll have ahead of time, and save a bottle cap, lime wedge, or swizzle stick from each. Studies have found that people

## # BY THE NUMBERS

**60** Number of fewer calories' worth of sugary snacks people eat later in the day when they chew sugar-free gum after lunch.

tend to consume less when they have a physical reminder of how much they've already had. And sip smarter: Anything served in a bottle will help you avoid bartender overpours. Most wines and light beers have about 100 to 125 calories per serving; if you want something stronger, try a Manhattan (130 calories), mojito (150), or vodka tonic (170).

## The Obstacle: Holiday Mentality

One reason a weekly routine helps is that you're more likely to stick to your chosen foods because it's easier. We tend to treat weekends like holidays—problem is, they come 52 times a year. That's a whole lot of Thanksgivings to get through. If sticking to your Monday-to-Friday routine sounds unfeasible, then a cheat meal can be helpful. When you allot yourself one cheat meal over the course of the weekend, you end up being more selective about your choices.

 **2-SECOND LIFE CHANGER**

***Open a window.*** Nothing smells as good as the scent of cinnamon and sugar wafting through your kitchen, but allowing the scent of home-baked holiday treats to linger for hours can trigger you to eat more. Crack a window to air out the tempting aroma.

## The Obstacle: Liquid Calories

Research shows that Americans drink an average of 458 calories every day—or more than one-fifth of our daily calorie intake. If that sounds like a lot, it is: In 1965, we drank just 236 calories daily. It's not just soda and cocktails: Even healthy beverages—like that 400-calorie pressed fruit and vegetable juice you picked up after your workout— can jack up your calorie count.

Get served a slimmer drink at your local coffee shop by using this calorie-cutting lingo.

**HOLD THE WHIP:** Cut the cream and save anywhere from 50 to 110 calories.

**ORDER IT FAT FREE:** Replace whole or 2% with fat-free milk.

**REQUEST SUGAR-FREE SYRUP:** Use instead of regular syrup and save up to 150 calories a drink.

**SAY "SKINNY":** Your drink will be made with sugar-free syrup and fat-free milk.

# The Obstacle: Movie Night

If you're too busy gazing at Ryan Gosling on the big screen, you're not focused on what you're eating. Sit down with a supersize popcorn, and before you know it, you just ate hundreds of calories. (That's no exaggeration: A *Consumer Reports* study found that the largest plain movie popcorn can have 1,269 calories and 81 grams of fat.) The best solution? Control what you put in front of you. Choose the smallest serving size available (researchers found that people tend to eat much more from large containers). Or sneak in your own healthy snack like a homemade trail mix.

 **SHAPE-UP SETBACK**

Here's a surprising diet shortcut that can help slash calories: Control your emotions to control your waistline. Researchers at the Miriam Hospital's Weight Control and Diabetes Research Center in Providence, Rhode Island, agree: They found that internal emotional triggers pose a larger obstacle to weight loss than external ones (say, for example, eating more because dinner is served buffet-style). Ending your day with a few cookies or a bowl of ice cream isn't the same as using them as your go-to stress-fighting strategy. Before you dive in, pause and ask yourself, "Why am I eating this?" If it's because you're angry, or sad, or upset, back away from the food and find another way to decompress, like taking a brisk walk, venting to a friend, or simply taking 10 super-slow breaths.

## The Obstacle: "I Don't Wanna Cook" Syndrome

It should come as no surprise that weekends are the most popular days for dining out, according to the National Restaurant Association. But research has also found that eating dinner out adds 144 calories to your daily intake. It may not seem like a lot, but if you also ate out for lunch, that's another 158 calories—plus, any away-from-home snacks tack on about 107 calories each.

 **SLIM-DOWN SECRET**

*Build a snack-free zone.* The sight and smell of food can cause the body to experience hunger, whether or not you actually have an appetite. Keep snacks away from your desk to avoid mindless munching. Out of sight (and smell), out of mind.

A study in the *Journal of the American Dietetic Association* found that people who were given the same snack, either whole or cut into halves, consumed half as much when eating the latter, possibly because they considered only the number of items (not the size of the items) they ate.

*"If you can't fly
then run
If you can't run
then walk
If you can't walk
then crawl
But whatever you do
you must keep
moving forward."*

—MARTIN LUTHER KING, JR.

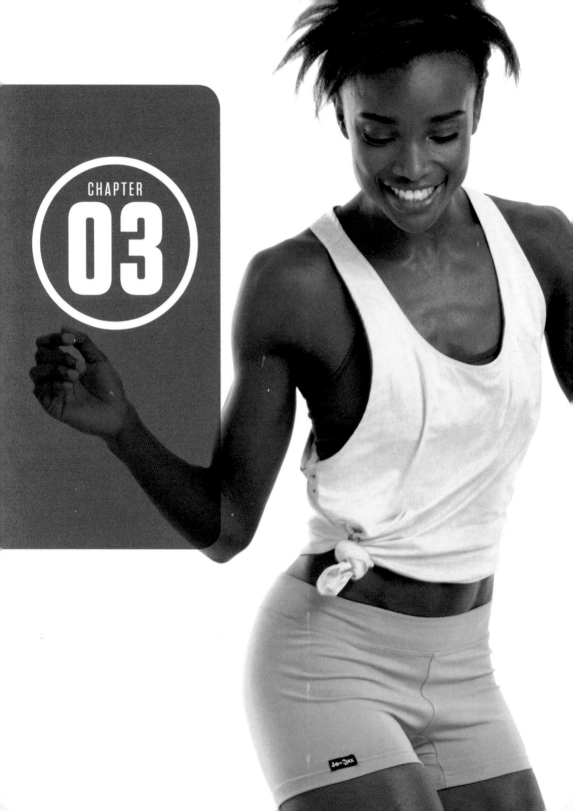

CHAPTER

# 03

# Upgrade
## Your
# Workout

*Spend less time in the gym—*
*and fast-track your results*

**O**ut of all the fitness myths, one of the most destructive is that you need to live at the gym to sculpt a strong, healthy, hot-looking body. That's because it has a polarizing effect: Some women reject a fitness routine altogether, either because they're too daunted to get started or they've tried and failed; others unknowingly push themselves beyond the point of progress. Women tell me all the time—with great pride—about their back-to-back spin classes, the boot camp where they did hundreds of crunches and lunges, or how they knocked out a cool 10-miler just for the heck of it.

Impressive? Absolutely. Effective? That depends on your goal. More often than not, these lengthy routines don't have a direct correlation to physical changes. And super-active women are still griping about stubborn belly fat, wishing to lose those last 5 pounds. The problem isn't with their effort, it's with their approach. (In fact, research shows that 97 percent of dieters regain the weight they lost, and experts suspect that the likely cause is their workout method.)

When you stop seeing results, your first instinct may be to stay on the treadmill longer, or add a hundred crunches to the end of every workout. But tacking on a few extra minutes won't rescue you from a plateau.—as your body adapts to a particular workout, it becomes more efficient and uses less energy (that is, you burn fewer calories).

Here's the good news: The secret to a hotter body is to sweat smarter, not harder, and, in many cases, for shorter durations. In fact, a study from McMaster University in Hamilton, Ontario, found that people who did brief, fast-paced workouts for a total of 90 minutes a week got just as fit as those who did lower-intensity training for 4 hours and 30 minutes. (Hello! That's an extra 3 hours a week!)

But not every short-and-sweet workout is created equal. This chapter is packed with smarter workout strategies and simple time-saving solutions to help you unleash your hottest body ever.

# Start Smarter

▶ Somewhere between lacing up your sneaks and starting your first set of squats, you face the most important decision of your workout: warm up or not? There's a good chance you just skip it. After all, you can barely carve out a 30-minute workout window. Who wants to waste even 1 valuable calorie-torching minute on tedious knee hugs and neck rolls?

But the short-term investment pays off big-time, even if the subsequent sweat session is only minutes long—as long as you do it right. The best approach involves dynamic stretching, which increases flexibility, improves blood flow, and decreases your risk of injury and recovery time. This means your workout will feel easier, and you'll see faster results.

Even better, warming up doesn't have to suck up a lot of time. In as few as 3 minutes, you can increase blood flow and range of motion, improve mental performance, and reduce the risk of injury, says Andrea Fradkin, PhD, an associate professor of exercise science at Bloomsburg University in Pennsylvania. Another reason to keep it short: A study in the *Journal of Applied Physiology* found that lengthy warmups can fatigue you, compromising your actual workout.

There are three crucial steps to an efficient, dynamic warmup. Pick one of the exercises from each section below and do them in order for a minute each. (Try to pick movements that mimic what you're about to do—leg swings before a run, walking lunges before strength training.)

## 1. Turn It On

Even if your brain is saying "Bring it!" your muscles aren't ready to work when you first hit the gym. Your central nervous system, which controls movement and activity, is basically in "power save" mode (blame it on a day at the desk). So before you jump into a workout, your brain needs to signal to your body that it's time for quick, explosive activity. These moves kick your nervous system into high gear by calling your coordination into action while raising your heart rate and body temperature. The result: Your muscles respond more effectively during your workout.

## ⇒ CROSS-OVER JUMPING JACKS

Stand with your feet more than hip-width apart and your arms straight out to your sides at shoulder height (A). Simultaneously cross your arms in front of your chest and jump your right leg in front of your left (B). Quickly reverse to return to the start. Repeat, crossing your left leg in front of your right. That's 1 rep.

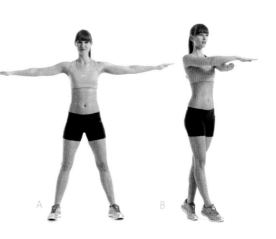

## ⇒ TIGHT CORE ROTATIONS

Stand with your feet more than hip-width apart and your arms extended in front of you, palms together (A). Keeping your hips and core engaged, rotate your upper body to the right (B). Quickly reverse, twisting all the way to the left. That's 1 rep.

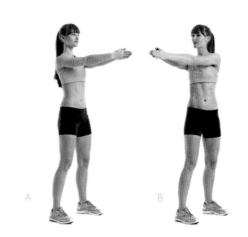

## ➡ HIGH SKIPS

Skip as high as you can by raising your right knee to hip height and simultaneously raising your left arm (A). Land on the ball of your left foot, then quickly repeat with your opposite arm and leg (B). That's 1 rep.

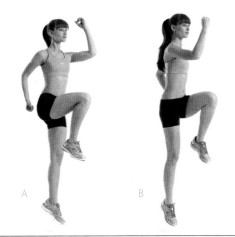

A          B

---

# 2. Up the Ante

Now that you've got your heart pumping, this phase will turn on weak and underused muscles: glutes, abdominals, hip flexors, and lower- and upper-back muscles. These "core muscles" are responsible for maintaining stability and control in your joints while you move. Forgetting to activate these muscles raises your risk of injury.

## ➡ SLOW-MOTION MOUNTAIN CLIMBER

Start at the top of a pushup (A). Keeping your abs braced, pick up your right foot and slowly bring your knee toward your right shoulder (B). Hold for 2 seconds, then return to the start. Alternate legs.

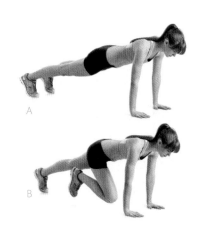

A

B

## ⇨ GLUTE BRIDGE MARCH

Lie on your back with your knees bent, feet flat on the floor. Raise your hips so your body forms a straight line from shoulders to knees (A). Brace your core and lift your right knee toward your chest (B). Hold for 2 counts, then lower your right foot. Repeat with the other leg. That's 1 rep.

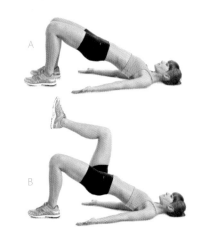

## ⇨ LEG OVERS

Lie faceup with your legs straight, arms at your sides (A). Sweep your right leg across your body toward your left hand, keeping your shoulders on the ground (B). Return to the start and switch legs. That's 1 rep.

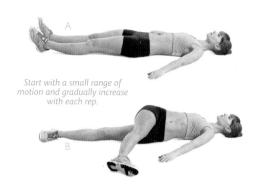

*Start with a small range of motion and gradually increase with each rep.*

# 3. Push Further

For the finale, you'll increase the range of motion at your joints, while improving the flexibility of your large muscle groups from head to toe (also known as dynamic mobility). And that's a big deal: When your mobility is compromised by stiff muscles, you spend more energy during your workout fighting against your body's limitations rather than burning calories.

## ➡ LOW LATERAL LUNGE

Step out to the right and bend your knee to lower into a side lunge, keeping your back flat and arms directly out in front of you (A). Without standing, shift to the left, into a lunge on the other side (B). That's 1 rep.

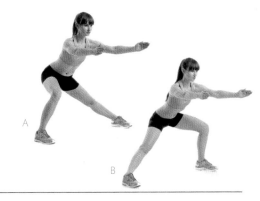

## ➡ SQUAT TO STAND

Stand with your feet shoulder-width apart. Keeping your legs straight, bend over and grab your toes. Without letting go of your toes, bend your knees to lower your body into a squat, raising your chest and shoulders (A). Holding that position, raise your left arm directly overhead (B), followed by your right (C). Press through your heels to rstand, then lower your arms. That's 1 rep.

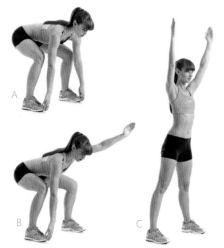

## ➡ REVERSE LUNGE WITH TWIST

Stand with your feet hip-width apart and your arms at your sides (A). In one mo-tion, step your left foot back and raise your arms overhead, bend both knees to lunge, as you twist your shoulders to the right (B). Reverse the movement to return to start. Repeat on the other side.

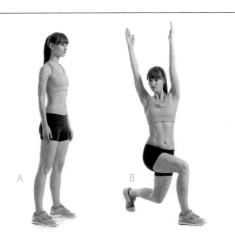

# Lose Your Fear of Lifting

➤ Think cardio is the key to blasting belly fat? Think again. Trade one or more of your weekly cardio workouts for a strength-training session to see faster waist-whittling results.

Lifting weights may be the single most efficient way to score a slimmer, sexier body. (In fact, a number of fitness pros suggest ditching traditional cardio altogether.) It also gives you an edge over belly fat, stress, heart disease, and cancer—and the list goes on and on. So why is it that, according to the *American Journal of Public Health*, only 16 percent of women meet the government's guideline for two or more strength-training sessions a week? These five prevalent myths may have something to do with it.

## Myth #1: Cardio burns more calories

For ages, many experts have said that calorie for calorie, aerobic exercise burns more calories than pumping iron. Not to mention, it *feels* true; not every trip to the weight room leaves you drenched and out of breath like a killer spin class (especially given that lifting newbies tend to have lower overall intensity, usually because they're hesitant). But it turns out that strength training has more calorie-torching potential than it was originally given credit for. Researchers at the University of Southern Maine found that completing a circuit of eight moves (which takes about 8 minutes) can expend 159 to 231 calories. This is about what you'd burn if you ran at a 10-mile-per-hour pace for the same duration.

In fact, the term *cardio* shouldn't be limited to only aerobic exercise: A study at the University of Hawaii found that circuit training with weights raises your heart rate 15 beats per minute higher than if you ran at 60 to 70 percent of your max heart rate. The circuit approach provides cardiovascular benefits similar to those of aerobic exercise while strengthening your muscles—so you save time without sacrificing results.

But here's where lifting really shines: Unlike aerobic exercise, the researchers found that a total-body workout with just three big-muscle moves raised participants' metabolisms for 39 hours afterward. Translation: Your body will continue to burn calories at a faster rate long after you've kicked off your sneakers. Sweet deal, right?

# Myth #2: You can outrun belly fat

This one's not even close: Weight training torches body fat better than hours of cardio. Plain and simple. In a study at the University of Alabama at Birmingham, one group of dieters lifted three times a week and another did aerobic exercise for the same amount of time. Both groups consumed the same number of calories, and both shed the same amount of weight (26 pounds). But those who pumped iron dropped 100 percent fat, whereas the cardio group lost 92 percent fat and 8 percent muscle. Here's why this matters: Muscle loss may drop your scale weight, but it doesn't improve your reflection in the mirror, and it makes you more likely to gain back the flab you lost. But if you strength-train while you diet, you'll build fat-fighting lean muscle mass and burn more fat. Experts estimate that for every 3 pounds of muscle you build, you can burn an extra 120 calories a day—just vegging—because muscle takes more energy to sustain. Over the course of a year, that's about 10 pounds of fat—without spending more time in the gym or changing your diet.

# Myth #3: Aerobic exercise keeps your heart healthy

Okay, yes, that's true, but cardio isn't the *only* way to get your blood pumping. Researchers at the University of Michigan found that people who did three total-body weight workouts a week for 2 months decreased their diastolic blood pressure (the bottom number) by an average of eight points. That's enough to reduce the risk of a stroke by 40 percent and the chance of a heart attack by 15 percent.

University of South Carolina researchers determined that total-body strength is linked to a lower risk of death from cardiovascular disease and cancer. Similarly, other scientists found that being strong during middle age is associated with "exceptional survival," defined as living to the age of 85 without developing a major disease.

# Myth #4: Lifting makes you bulky

I receive pitches and reviews every day of new workout methods that create "long and lean muscles." I hear ladies say they don't lift because they're looking to get "toned," not "bulky." We even use it in the magazine as a way of describing the overall aesthetic many of our readers are trying to achieve.

But here's some news that might disappoint a lot of women—and even more trainers who play into the female fear of looking like the Hulk: Muscles, by definition, are lean; and their length is set once our body is mature. No workout can make them more lean, and, outside of surgery, there is not much that can permanently alter their length. In fact, there are only two ways that muscle can change its appearance: It can get bigger or get smaller.

This battle of toning versus bulking actually has nothing to do with the muscles themselves—it comes down to your overall body fat. This idea of looking toned is often an attempt to describe a body with a low enough body fat percentage to reveal muscle definition. When you build muscle, but don't attack the body fat that lies on top of it, you may feel bigger, heavier. Conversely, methods like Pilates and yoga typically don't use the same level of resistance, which may mean you're not building as much muscle; so even if your body fat percentage remains the same, you at least don't *feel* like you're getting denser. At the same time, many of these routines help improve posture, which can give the appearance that you are, in fact, "longer and leaner."

These light-resistance methods can actually sabotage your goals in the long run, though. Research shows that between the ages of 30 and 50, you'll likely lose 10 percent of your body's total muscle. Worse yet, it's likely to be replaced by fat over time, according to a study in the *American Journal of Clinical Nutrition*. Even participants who maintained their body weight for up to 38 years lost 3 pounds of muscle and added 3 pounds of fat every decade.

Why does that matter? Because even if their body weight remained the same, their pant size likely didn't. Not only does it help stoke your internal calorie burner, but lean muscle mass actually takes up 18 percent less space than 1 pound of fat. So to recap: Building lean muscle mass through strength training is the real secret to revealing a leaner, more toned body.

## Myth #5: To run better, you must run more

Practice makes perfect, right? Turns out, extra pavement pounding isn't the only—or necessarily the most effective—strategy. A review of studies in the *Journal of Strength and Conditioning Research* found that runners who did resistance-training exercises 2 or 3 days a week, in addition to their weekly cardio regimens, increased their leg strength and enhanced their endurance—two things that improve performance and contribute to weight loss.

Lifting can also keep you injury free: A study in the journal *Clinical Biomechanics* found that female runners who did 6 weeks of lower-body exercises improved their leg strength, particularly in the hips—a common source of pain and injury for runners.

# WHERE'S THE CARDIO?

## Don't get me wrong: I love running.

It's a workout that ignites a surge of endorphins—chemicals your brain releases during exercise—making your hard work feel good. I spent many years of my athletic life viewing running as merely a means to an end. The miles I logged were just a way to make sure I was ready to hit the field. But, in the past few years, I've learned to enjoy the satisfaction that comes from running as the only objective. Crossing the line of two half-marathons and a triathlon, I felt a rush of accomplishment and excitement—and I instantly understood the attraction.

But here's why you won't find tons of talk about running (or cycling, or swimming) in this chapter: It's not the most efficient way to burn calories and body fat. (And it's not the only way to get that feel-good high.) Like I mentioned earlier, the term *cardio* has always seemed interchangeably linked to aerobic training, but it actually stands for "cardiovascular exercise"—or an activity that raises your heart rate to 60 to 85 percent of its max. By way of design, the majority of the workouts you'll find in this book count as cardio training. That said, we'll take a closer look at the specifics of aerobic exercise in Chapter 7.

# Ditch the Machines

➤ You spend a lot of time sitting each day—at work, in the car, on the couch. But in the weight room?

Free weights, such as barbells and dumbbells, challenge your body more than machines do, according to a study in the *Journal of Strength and Conditioning Research*. They engage more muscles, increase range of motion, and are less likely to cause injury. Still, many women spend the majority of their time at the gym hopping from one exercise machine to the next. The problem: "Many machines isolate one muscle, which means you burn fewer calories and work fewer muscles," says Mike Boyle, owner of Mike Boyle Strength & Conditioning in Woburn and North Andover. Next time you hit the gym, sub in these replacement exercises instead.

**THE MACHINE:**
## SEATED LEG EXTENSION

Sure, you'll strengthen your quads—but at a cost. The resistance is close to your ankle, which puts a high amount of torque on your knee when you raise and lower the weight, says Boyle. The result? Kneecap pain.

**THE REPLACEMENT:**
## SPLIT SQUAT

This move puts less stress on your knees, plus it works your hamstrings and glutes. Step one foot 3 to 4 feet in front of the other (A), then bend your knees and lower your back knee toward the floor (B). Press through the heel of the front foot to stand. Do 10 reps, then switch legs and repeat.

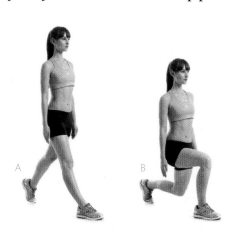

A          B

# SEATED ABS CRUNCH

Simply put, spinal flexion (the act of bending forward as you do during a crunch) is the cause of most adult back pain, says Boyle. Think of it like a credit card: "Bend the card once and it probably won't break. But bend it 100 times and see what happens." And, by adding weight, this machine places even more pressure on your spinal discs, increasing the risk of pain and injury.

**THE REPLACEMENT:**

# STABILITY-BALL ROLLOUT

Your core is meant to stabilize your spine, not move it, and this exercise engages your entire core to keep your spine neutral. Kneel on the ground and place your forearms on a stability ball, palms together (A). Brace your core and slowly roll the ball away from you, keeping your back flat (B). Slowly pull the ball back to the starting position. That's 1 rep. Work up to 20.

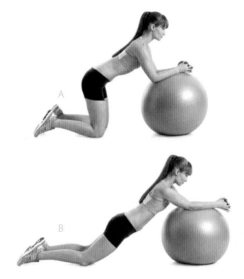

**THE MACHINE:**

# HIP ADDUCTOR/ABDUCTOR

Sitting down and squeezing your legs together or pushing them apart won't shrink your thighs no matter how many reps you bang out. "These are nonfunctional, unnatural movement patterns that offer zero payoff," says Boyle. And the abductor move could irritate your iliotibial band, the ropey piece of connective tissue that runs from the outside of your hip to the outside of your knee.

# PLIÉ SQUAT

Pliés are a far better leg toner because they hit your inner thighs and your quads, hamstrings, and glutes. Stand with your feet wide and turned out 45 degrees (A). Sit your hips back and bend your knees to lower your body until your thighs are nearly parallel to the floor (B). Return to the start. That's 1 rep. Do 3 sets of 10.

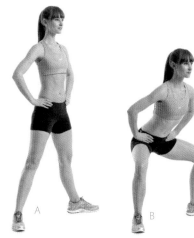

# LATERAL BAND WALK

Lateral band walks tone the outer thighs, glutes, and hips. Place a small resistance loop above your ankles and sidestep to the right for 15 feet. Step to the left to return to the starting position. That's 1 set. Repeat 2 more times.

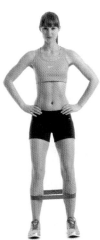

# BICEPS CURL

The biggest problem here is that it's so easy to cheat! People often rely on gravity to lower (read: drop) the bar, and cutting your range of motion short not only makes the exercise less effective, but also causes muscle tightness and strains your elbows and wrists.

## ➡ BAND-ASSISTED CHINUP

This move hits your biceps, back, shoulders, and core, and strengthens the muscles that help you stand tall, so you look longer and leaner. Loop a resistance band around a chinup bar, threading one end through the other and pulling it tightly. Grab the bar with a shoulder-width, underhand grip, place your knee in the loop of the band, and hang at arm's length (A). Pull yourself up to the bar (B). Work up to 10 reps.

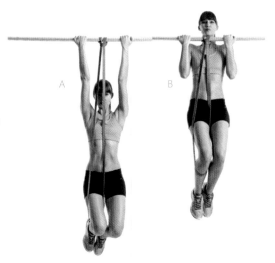

# Fix Your Form

➤ If you've been going to the gym regularly and not seeing great results, it may be because you're unknowingly mangling your moves (no offense). Experts agree that proper form is the single most important factor in injury prevention, yet many women don't give it a lot of thought—especially when they're in a rush.

The truth is, most people make tiny but key errors in their techniques, and these mistakes prevent them from building muscle and burning more calories. The four basic moves on the next two pages have a tendency to trip women up. Apply these form fixes to upgrade your routine—and your body.

*Quick tip: A good strategy for first-timers: Do all the exercises without any resistance. Going through the movement pattern with proper form—but no heavy weights—helps teach your body and brain how to move.*

# ⇒ LUNGES

**MAIN MISTAKE:** You lean forward, causing your front heel to rise.

Narrow your starting stance. The closer your feet are, the harder your core has to work to stabilize your body (A).

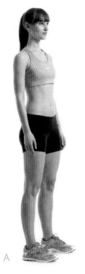

As you do the lunge, focus on moving your torso only up and down, not pushing it forward. This keeps your weight balanced evenly through your front foot, allowing you to press into the floor with your heel, which tones more lower-body muscles (B).

*Drop your back knee straight down to the floor.*

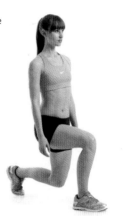

A

B

---

# ⇒ SQUATS

**MAIN MISTAKE:** You start the movement by bending your knees.

Women tend to lean forward on their toes, but they should sit back into their heels. Try this fix: Pretend that you're standing on a paper towel and imagine trying to rip the towel apart by pressing your feet onto the floor and outward (A). This activates your glutes, which helps you break through plateaus.

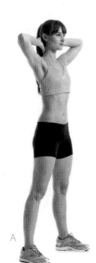

As you squat, imagine you're sitting down into a chair, rather than forward on top of your knees. Push your hips back first instead of beginning by bending your knees, which puts more stress on your joints (B).

*As you stand, think about pushing the floor away from your body, rather than lifting your body.*

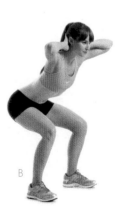

A

B

# STRAIGHT-LEG DEADLIFTS

**MAIN MISTAKE:** You round your lower back as you bend over.

It's easy to put too much space between the weight and your body as you move up and down. Pretend you're shaving your legs with the bar or dumbbells. The farther the weights are from your body, the more strain on your back, which limits the work of your hamstrings and glutes.

When bending down, act as if you are holding a tray of drinks and need to close the door behind you with your backside (A).

This helps you push your hips back instead of rounding your lower back—a form blunder that puts you at risk for back problems.

As you return to standing, squeeze your glutes. You'll engage your butt rather than strain your lower back (B).

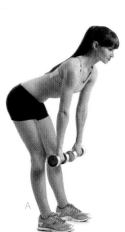

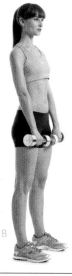

A

B

# ROWS AND PULLUPS

**MAIN MISTAKE:** You ignore the muscles that draw back your shoulder blades.

Before you start the exercise, create as much space as you can between your ears and shoulders. Pull your shoulder blades down and back, which will ensure you work the intended middle- and upper-back muscles (A).

Imagine there is an orange between your shoulder blades. As you pull the weights or your body up, "squeeze the juice out of it" by bringing your shoulder blades together (B).

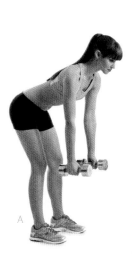

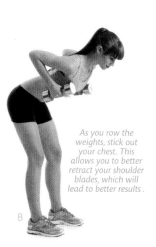

*As you row the weights, stick out your chest. This allows you to better retract your shoulder blades, which will lead to better results.*

A

B

# CHANGE UP YOUR GRIP

You often hear that your hands should be shoulder-width apart for upper-body moves like pushups, bench presses, and lat pull-downs. Why? Because it gives you a stable starting point. This doesn't mean it's the only option. Spreading your hands a few inches farther out engages more of the inner portion of your biceps; bringing your hands in a few inches builds more of the outer part. Here are three basic grips you'll see in various workouts throughout this book. They may seem like subtle changes, but they make a big difference: With a flick of the wrists, you can engage different muscles.

| *Neutral grip* | *Overhand grip* | *Underhand grip* |
|---|---|---|
| Palms facing each other. | Palms facing down or back. Also called a pronated grip. | Palms facing up or forward. Also called a reverse grip or supinated grip. |

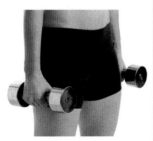 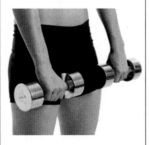 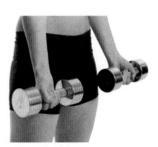

# Burn Fat Faster

You've already read about how turning up the intensity on your workout can help slash pounds—and time spent at the gym. And while it's relatively easy to translate higher intensity into spin class (pedal faster) or on the treadmill (dial up the pace), many women aren't sure how exactly to best increase efforts during their strength-training workouts. Fast-track your results by incorporating the following training strategies.

## Watch Your Speed

If you think pace only matters when you're out on a run, think again: The speed of your resistance training matters, too. But it may be one of the most overlooked building blocks to an effective strength-training routine.

In the weight room, tempo training refers to the speed you lift and lower resistance during an exercise, and adjusting it is a great way to get more out of every rep. Sometimes this means moving through exercises more quickly: Researchers at Anderson University and Ball State University in Indiana found that exercisers who performed a weight-lifting workout at a quick, explosive pace

# STEADY AT ANY SPEED

Regardless of what tempo you're moving at, one thing should stay the same: You never want to train at a speed that compromises control. When any workout cranks up the intensity or speed, quality can take a backseat to quantity. People sometimes get so focused on banging out as many reps as they can, however they can—even if it means sacrificing form. While the occasional slam of a weight stack is par for the course when using resistance equipment like the cable machine, lowering the weight without control can result in injury. It can also prevent you from getting the results you're after, because you don't work through the full range of motion. With every exercise, make sure your primary objective is proper form—then you can worry about tempo.

expended 70 more calories, on average, than those who did the workout at a normal pace.

You can also score benefits from slowing down your workouts. Your muscle has three main types of contractions: eccentric (lengthening of muscle fibers during the lowering portion of an exercise, like lowering into a squat), isometric (muscle length staying the same while under tension, like the bottom position of a squat), and concentric (the shortening of muscle fibers during the lifting portion of the exercise, like standing up from a squat). Slowing down during the eccentric portion of an exercise can help improve body awareness and stability, as well as stimulate the muscle fibers differently by placing them under more stress. The *Journal of Strength and Conditioning Research* found that an eccentric tempo (taking 3 seconds) significantly increased the amount of calories that both trained and untrained individuals burned for up to 72 hours post-workout. The slow eccentric phase increases the tension on the muscle, which creates a higher calorie burn during and after exercise in order to repair the muscles.

And, yes, you can even burn calories without moving a muscle. It's called isometric training, after that second muscle contraction where the muscle length stays the same while under tension. Take a wall squat, for example: Your quads are constantly under stress, even though they don't move. This can be an especially useful strategy for people who lack stability or are dealing with injuries.

# WEIGH YOUR OPTIONS

**Lifting too much too soon** can hurt your form and put you at risk for injury, but grabbing 2-pounders won't test your muscles enough to yield results. Use this cheat sheet to gauge starting weights for beginners.

| If you're doing . . . | Start with . . . |
|---|---|
| lateral raises | 2½ to 5 pounds in each hand |
| biceps curls | 5 to 8 pounds in each hand |
| flat-bench dumbbell rows | 12 to 20 pounds |
| chest presses | 12 pounds (body bar) to 45 pounds |
| squats | zero (body weight) to 45 pounds |

Like other pieces of your workout program, you should mix up tempos so your body doesn't adapt to the pace.

## Lift Heavy

Dumbbells, resistance bands, even water—they're all ways to apply external force to your workout to make any routine more challenging. The added stress encourages muscle growth, which helps increase your metabolism and blast fat. But in order to get a tighter, leaner body, the chosen resistance has to actually tax your muscles.

This means saying goodbye to feather-light dumbbells. I'm not saying that lifting lighter weights is completely ineffective. Researchers found that lifting 30 percent of your all-out max can be as effective as 80 percent of your max—but, here's the important part—as long as you do enough reps to tire out your muscles. Translation: It's going to take considerably more reps at a lighter weight to match the effectiveness. But, again, it comes

 **SHAPE-UP SETBACK**

Don't even think about skipping the last few reps—this is where the magic happens, so to speak. You have to stress your muscles if you want them to change, and that occurs in those last few reps of the exercise. Your last reps should be tough to finish, but not so difficult that you have to compromise your form. And if you're busting out 15 to 20 reps with no trouble at all, it's time to increase the challenge—by adding more weight or performing a more difficult exercise.

back to your goal. If it is faster fat loss, supersizing your dumbbells is a better use of your gym time. Hoisting heavier weights builds lean muscle in less time, plus research shows you can burn nearly twice as many calories in the 2 hours after lifting heavier weights.

# Use More Muscle

Many women, especially if they're new to strength training, stick to a handful of the same exercises (things like biceps curls, calf raises, and crunches). They eventually work a good amount of muscles, head to toe, but it takes a while since they're only focusing on one muscle group at a time, known as isolation exercises.

 **SLIM-DOWN SECRET**

People lost two times more fat when they trained their entire body 3 days a week, compared to working each muscle group only once a week, according to University of Alabama scientists.

When you listen to some of the top sports performance coaches in the country—Mike Robertson, Eric Cressey, and Mike Boyle are just a few names that come to mind—their opinions have a familiar theme: Even if the end goal is simply to look great in a bikini, women would benefit from a more athletic training approach. The strength work of athletes places a significant emphasis on movements that we replicate in real life—like squatting, pushing, stepping, jumping, and pulling—rather than just body parts or single muscle groups. Also referred to as "functional training," these big-body exercises help you move bigger weights and build more muscle. At the same time, this movement-centered approach improves mobility, meaning your muscles and joints are able to withstand the stress placed on them during workouts and throughout each day without getting injured.

But you won't just move better and feel stronger: Targeting multiple muscle groups at once (called compound exercises) recruits more muscle fibers, which translates to a higher calorie burn in less time. This functional approach also makes your body a stronger, more efficient unit, so you can challenge it more (read: work it harder and see results faster). Take a look at your workout; no less than 50 percent of the exercises should be big-body moves, as opposed to isolated (or single-joint) exercises.

## Rest Less

If you walk into any weight room, you'll likely find a handful of people standing around not doing much that resembles working out. I can still remember spending up to an hour at a time in my high-school weight room over the summer to prepare for field hockey preseason. I used to think that made me sound impressive, but I probably spent 70 percent

 **2-SECOND LIFE CHANGER**

You can save even more time during supersets by pairing noncompeting muscle groups (think upper and lower body). So while your arms take a break from biceps curls, your legs can get busy doing squats—which means fewer, and even shorter, rest breaks.

of the time sitting around "resting" between sets, and watching all the football players do the same. It was tedious and slow, and certainly didn't feel like the most effective workout.

Way back then, I overlooked a crucial point: Just because my legs needed a break after squats didn't mean my whole body did. With the right program, you can take advantage of that downtime by training another muscle group. Take supersets: two exercises that work opposing muscle groups, performed back to back without rest—for example, a chest press combined with a bent-over row. Supersets accomplish more work in a shorter period of time without compromising the effort of each set. In fact, a study in the *Journal of Strength and Conditioning Research* found that participants burned 33 percent more calories after doing supersets compared with sets that let you rest between moves.

Another popular method: circuit training. This is when you move through a series of strength exercises, going from one to the next with little to no rest. It's a simple shortcut that cuts your gym time in half, without cutting corners on your results. What's more, minimizing your downtime between moves also keeps your heart rate elevated and helps maximize the fat-burning impact of your workout. And you know

# PUSH YOUR LIMITS

Who doesn't dig spa days, calming yoga sessions, and Sunday sleep-ins? But when it comes to short-and-sweet workouts, your comfort may need to take a backseat.

Researchers at McMaster University found that exercising as hard as you can for short periods of time is just as effective at improving muscle and metabolism as sweating it out longer at a lower intensity. The Tabata method, for example, involves fast-and-furious intervals—20 seconds of all-out effort followed by 10 seconds of rest—repeated a total of eight times. That's a whopping 4 minutes.

Problem is, without someone egging you on, you may hit the brakes as soon as your workout gets the slightest bit uncomfortable (unlike the study participants, who were killing it during 30-second intervals). When it comes to high-intensity effort, you have to force your body past the point of wanting to quit—a point trainers call volitional fatigue, or when you can't do another rep with perfect form.

Sound intense? Well, that's the point. But just remember: In less than half an hour, you'll be done and hitting the shower. And in a few months from now, when you're slipping into a smaller dress size or confidently rocking a tiny two-piece, it will have been totally worth it.

what's more impressive than spending an hour in the weight room? Spending only 30 minutes—and getting an even better workout.

## Power Up

Muscle strength isn't the only thing that can jump-start a sluggish metabolism. Muscle power (sometimes referred to as speed-strength by trainers) is about generating as much force as fast as possible, and it can be a useful weight-loss tool.

In fact, workouts that incorporate explosive movements, commonly referred to as plyometrics, are one of the most effective ways to torch calories and burn serious fat. They also fire up your fitness level by improving your coordination and agility. They can even boost your speed: Researchers at the University of Nebraska found that participants who improved their vertical jump also logged significantly faster 10-K running times.

Whether they're jumps or quick upper-body movements, plyometric exercises increase the elastic properties of your muscles, which, over time, allows them to handle intense workloads more efficiently. The result: Your muscles adapt to more challenging workouts faster, so you see body-shaping results sooner.

Because these types of exercises can be higher impact and harder on your joints, ease into them slowly; when starting a new plyo routine, do it only once a week for the first 2 weeks.

 **SLIM-DOWN SECRET**

Don't even open the door to the gym unless you have a clear plan in mind. You'll likely end up wandering around, wasting time, and not trying all that hard. Figure out what equipment you need—dumbbells, stability ball, bands—and put it near a mat or adjustable bench so you can do your entire workout in one place. Bonus: By creating your own personal space at the gym, you maximize your intensity and efficiency, keeping your heart rate and metabolism up the entire time by moving from one exercise to the next.

# Body by You

➥ No costly memberships, no sweaty strangers, no stressing to get there before it closes—it's no big surprise that people with home gyms were 73 percent more likely to be active than those without one. But you don't need a ton of equipment to get into great shape. Here are a few of the best pieces to bring home.

## DUMBBELLS

There's nothing glitzy about them, but dumbbells are the single most essential workout tool to keep around. There are literally hundreds of exercises you can do with them. If you can, get at least two pairs (one light, one heavy) so that you can switch them up depending on the exercise. I like Perform Better Rubber Encased Dumbbells at performbetter.com.

### 2-SECOND LIFE CHANGER

Research shows that plyometrics may also be the key to stronger bones. Your bones constantly go through a rebuilding process to maintain a healthy density. And the best way to trigger that rebuilding is by stressing them with explosive movements, according to a review in *Sports Medicine*. Bone density peaks between ages 25 and 30, and then decreases by 1 to 2 percent a year, so the higher your bone density is before it begins thinning, the lower your risk for osteoporosis later on.

## CHINUP BAR

Bodyweight exercises cover every basic movement—except pulling. Nothing trains you better than classic chinups. You can find a number of at-home, removable options, like Gold's Gym Multi-Training Door Gym at getgoldsgym.com.

## FOAM ROLLER

Soothe sore muscles and loosen tight fascia (the connective tissue that surrounds muscles) for improved recovery, better performance, and a more lithe look. There are endless options, but I like having a full-length roller (like Black Axis Firm Foam Roller, at optp.com) and a smaller, more portable option (like Trigger Point Grid Mini, tptherapy.com).

## SLIM-DOWN SECRET

Training with a partner can simultaneously motivate and distract you during a tough workout, which can help you score better results. A study from the University of Pittsburgh reports that women who joined a weight-loss program with a pal lost one-third more weight than those who went solo. But there's a subtle—and crucial—aspect to the approach that's often overlooked: Not any workout buddy will do; it has to be one who will push you. While you may love running with a girlfriend who clocks a slower per-mile pace, sticking with her isn't doing you any good. Being the underdog in a running or CrossFit workout group will only make you stronger.

## VALSLIDE

These sliding discs increase the friction of almost any surface—turning your hardwood floor, carpet, or tile into a skating rink. The result: Your muscles are under constant tension during every exercise, which boosts the effectiveness. You can find them at valslide.com. (Find a Valslide workout on page 186.)

## STABILITY BALL

It's a great tool for core exercises and can also substitute for a bench in some exercises to increase the difficulty and up the core activation. The Gymnic Classic Plus Exercise Ball at optp.com is just one of numerous choices.

## TRX

This suspension trainer leverages your own weight to adjust the resistance of any total-body move. Setup is simple—just flip over a door or around a (sturdy) stair banister—and it packs into a small bag so you can stash it when you're not using it. Find the TRX Home suspension trainer at trxtraining.com.

## RESISTANCE BANDS

Big ones (like Superbands at performbetter.com) can make bodyweight squats extra challenging or help with assisted chinups, while smaller bands (I love GoFit Power Loops 3-pack from gofit.net) are one of my favorite tools for waking up the underworked muscles in your hips and butt.

## KETTLEBELL

It can be used in the same way as dumbbells, but because of its unique shape, it's even more versatile. (Find the Ultimate Lean-Body Kettlebell Workout on page 168.) You can find great options at power-systems.com or performbetter.com.

## JUMP ROPE

For just a few bucks you can have a portable, calorie-incinerating tool that's perfect for picking up your heart rate during a warmup, or spiking your calorie-burn totals during your workout.

## BENCH, STEP, OR BOX

Adjustable benches add variety to free-weight training; a basic cardio step or box can be a great starting point for beginners.

# Stop Playing Favorites

⬛ Here's one gym shortcut you never want to take: selective strength training. The ever-popular philosophy known as "spot reducing" is a shortcut dieter's dream: It states that if you exercise a specific muscle group, you'll burn fat in that area. Don't love your thighs? Just keep lunging and they'll get leaner. Trying to lose your belly? Bang out enough crunches and the fat will melt right off.

Sound too good to be true? That's because it is. Fat and muscle are two completely independent tissues. Training every day with endless

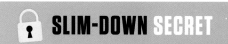

**SLIM-DOWN SECRET**

People who pushed themselves in the first half of a workout and eased up during the second half burned 23 percent more fat than those who did the opposite, according to a study from the College of New Jersey in Ewing.

crunches and planks will strengthen those muscles, but it won't directly impact the fat surrounding them to flatten your belly faster. To reveal a tight, flat stomach, you need to build more lean muscle *all over*, which increases your metabolic rate (the number of calories you burn daily) and helps you shed stubborn body fat faster.

But there's also a subtler variation of spot reduction—something I like to

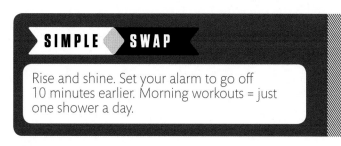

**SIMPLE ▶ SWAP**

Rise and shine. Set your alarm to go off 10 minutes earlier. Morning workouts = just one shower a day.

call wish-list workouts. Instead of zeroing in on a single muscle group, they choose exercises that target a few areas—like, say, triceps, abs, and thighs. On the surface, this looks (and probably feels) like a total-body workout. And yes, it increases your body's fat-burning potential because you're engaging a higher percentage of muscle fibers compared to training only one muscle. But working out this way might neglect some crucial supporting players and create muscular imbalances, which can have a big impact on your results.

# BALANCING ACT

## Improve your selective approach with these three tips.

### Turn around.
Women have a tendency to focus on "mirror muscles." For every exercise that works the front of the body (chest, biceps, quads), be sure to do an exercise that targets the rear (back, triceps, hamstrings).

### Scale back.
Train your abs 3 days a week—that's it. Stressing your muscles during a workout breaks down the tissues, and they need rest days to rebuild and get stronger. You'll see benefits quicker and prevent injury if you stick to three sessions a week (on nonconsecutive days).

### Play favorites.
There is a way to give certain areas a little more love. A lot of people squeeze in selective strength training after their workouts—like a few hundred crunches after a spin class. But that's when you get sloppy or run out of time. Do abs work first, and then move on to the rest of the workout .

# Create Perfect Balance

Nearly every major muscle group in your body has a corresponding group that carries out the opposite function. Take your biceps and triceps: Their even matchup lets you bend and straighten your elbow without any thought. At least, that's how it should work.

Unfortunately, everyday habits (like sitting at a desk), repetitive workouts (say, that marathon you're training for or your three-times-a-week spin class), and even your wardrobe (pointing at those skyscraper heels) threaten these partnerships. The result: One of the muscles becomes stronger and overpowers the other, a common condition known as muscular imbalance.

Like any team, if one area is weak, another part must pick up the slack, and the entire system suffers. The danger of muscular imbalances is that they alter your nat-

 **2-SECOND LIFE CHANGER**

Doing cardio before resistance training zaps strength and energy levels fast, so save it for the end of your routine. And, if you're running out of time, don't worry about the clock, just go harder. You'll improve your conditioning more by running at a higher intensity for 15 minutes than with a slow 30-minute jog.

ural movement patterns. Over time, they can pull bones and joints out of alignment, which often leads to pain and injury.

They can also worsen poor posture and wreak havoc on your figure. (Tight hip flexors, for example, can tilt your hips forward and give the look of a stomach pooch.) Correcting imbalances helps elongate your silhouette and can make you look 5 pounds lighter.

The fix isn't as simple as isolating the pair and strengthening the weak muscle while leaving the other alone. That's because muscles, ligaments, tendons, and bones are all connected and dependent on each other through an intricate system—known by trainers and doctors as the kinetic chain. This system relies on the cooperation of two interrelated principles to promote movement throughout your body: stability, which allows muscles, tendons, and ligaments to hold a joint in position; and mobility, which permits both the joint to safely move through a full range of motion and the nearby muscles to cause that motion. Because the collection of parts functions as a whole, when one of those elements is lacking in one area of the body, it throws off the rest of your body. Meaning, your back pain could actually stem from a problem with your shoulder, your knee, or even your shin.

That said, knowing what imbalances you may have can help ID what's causing your pain—and spotting them early can mean preventing future injuries. Here are simple self-tests on three common female imbalances. If an area is out of whack, work the fix into your total-body routine at least three times a week.

# Chest versus Back

A balanced upper body helps you stand taller, look leaner, and stave off shoulder and back pain. Problem is, many women prioritize their arms and abs over their back and chest. Combined with spending hours hunched over a keyboard, this imbalance can cause what experts call a protracted shoulder girdle (what you know as rounded shoulders and slouchy posture). It's a sign that the muscles on the front of your body are tight, while your back muscles are weak.

**TEST IT:**
Lie faceup with your arms by your sides, palms facing in. Raise your arms overhead until they touch the floor. If your back arches, your palms turn toward the ceiling, your elbows point outward, or you can't touch your arms to the floor, you need to improve this imbalance.

**FIX IT:**
## LYING DUMBBELL PULLOVER

Lie faceup on a bench, feet flat on the floor, holding a pair of dumbbells directly over your chest, arms completely straight (A). Keeping your arms straight, brace your core and lower the weights toward the floor as far as you can, or until your arms are in line with your ears (B). Pause, then raise the weights back to the start. That's 1 rep. Do 10 to 12.

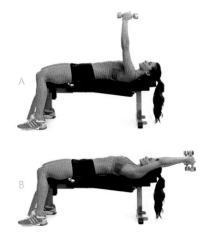

# Quadriceps versus Hamstrings

Out of the biological gate, women are more likely to be quad dominant (meaning they use their quads more than their hamstrings) than men are. Wider hips throw off lower-body alignment and make it difficult for the posterior muscles, like your hamstrings, to work properly. It's made worse by thigh-centric workout programs that emphasize the quads—two of many women's go-to lower-body moves are lunges and squats.

Striking a more even balance can lower your risk for injury as well as increase your running speed and overall power. A study in the *American Journal of Sports Medicine* found that 70 percent of athletes with recurring hamstring injuries suffered from muscle imbalances between their quadriceps and hamstrings. After correcting the imbalances by strengthening the hamstrings, every person in the study went injury free for the entire year after.

**TEST IT:**

Stand in front of a chair that's a foot away from a wall, your toes 6 inches from the wall, feet hip-width apart, and arms raised overhead. Keeping your arms overhead and chest upright, squat into the chair. If you lose your balance, raise your heels off the floor, or touch the wall, you likely have dominant quads.

**FIX IT:**

## STABILITY BALL LEG CURL

Lie on the floor with your calves on a stability ball (A). Raise your hips, then pull the ball toward you (B). Return to the start. That's 1 rep. Do 10 to 12.

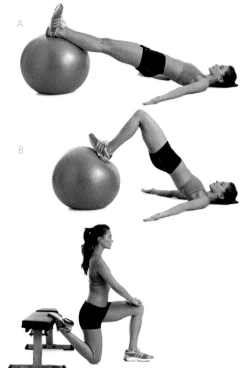

## KNEELING QUAD STRETCH

Kneel in front of a step or bench, placing one foot flat on the floor in front of you. Raise your back foot and place it against the step or bench. Hold for 15 to 20 seconds, then switch sides and repeat.

# Glutes versus Hip Flexors

Your glute muscles are the powerhouse of your lower half, plus they help stabilize your hips and pelvis, keeping your spine properly aligned. Yet, most people don't train them nearly as much as they should. What's more, over time, sitting around too much causes your glutes to lose strength and eventually even forget how to contract (or as *Women's Health* fitness expert Rachel Cosgrove says, develop "gluteal amnesia"). At the same time, your hip flexors—the muscles that connect your hip bones to your legs—become short and stiff. This couch-potato combo tilts your pelvis forward, which increases the arch in your back and puts stress on your spine. From a cosmetic standpoint, it pushes your abdomen out, making even a relatively flat stomach bulge.

**TEST IT:**

Lie on a bench, knees at your chest. Holding one knee, lower the other leg as far as possible while keeping it straight. Switch legs. If either leg doesn't rest on the bench, you likely have tight hip flexors (a sign of weak glutes).

**FIX IT:**

## GLUTE BRIDGE

Lie faceup with your knees bent, feet flat on the floor (A). Raise your hips toward the ceiling (B); pause, then lower. That's 1 rep. Do 12 to 15.

A

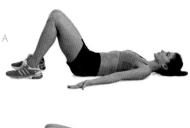

B

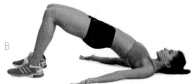

*If your hamstrings cramp up during the glute bridge, it could be a sign that your glutes are weak and your hamstrings are having to work extra hard to keep your hips raised off the ground. Get your butt in gear by holding each rep for 3 to 5 seconds.*

## SCORPION

Lie facedown on the floor with your legs straight (A). Raise your right foot off the ground, bending your knee, and reach your toe to the left, lifting your right hip off the ground while keeping your upper body still (B). Hold for 3 seconds, then slowly reverse the movement to return to the start; that's 1 rep. Repeat on the other side and continue alternating for 10 to 12 total reps.

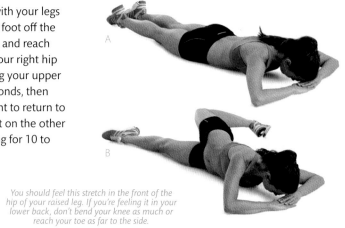

*You should feel this stretch in the front of the hip of your raised leg. If you're feeling it in your lower back, don't bend your knee as much or reach your toe as far to the side.*

*"Just as your car runs smoothly and requires less energy to run faster and farther when the wheels are in alignment, you perform better when your thoughts, feelings, emotions, goals, and values are in balance."*

—BRIAN TRACY

# THE COST OF HIGH HEELS

**Your high-heel habit** comes at a price. For starters, wearing them shifts your weight forward, placing more stress on your quads and less on your hamstrings and glutes (which doesn't help the imbalance you just read about). Plus, when you elevate the heels chronically, your ankle mobility—your toe-to-shin range of motion—suffers. This might not sound like a big deal, but it can actually cause a number of problems further up the kinetic chain.

It can also lead to a muscular imbalance between your calf and shin muscles. Strong shin muscles may not get you noticed in short shorts, but this small muscle is critical for controlling your foot landing. When it's weak, your calf muscles must absorb the extra shock, which can lead to shin splints. Wearing high heels makes it worse: Women who wore 2-inch heels (or higher) for at least 40 hours a week for at least 2 years walked differently than those who usually wore flats, according to a study in the *Journal of Applied Physiology*. If the foot is forced into a position in which the toes point downward, the shin muscles get weaker, calf muscles get shorter, and the Achilles tendon gets stiffer, which could lead to injuries over time.

## Fix It

*Stretch your calves.* Researchers found that people who sprain their ankles don't have the same range of motion in those joints as folks whose ankles stay injury free. Tight gastrocnemius and soleus muscles limit ankle motion.

*Take a break.* If you can, only wear towering heels once or twice a week, and kick them off while sitting at your desk.

*Add toe raises.* Using a chair for balance, slowly raise your toes off the ground; slowly lower them. That's 1 rep. Do 15 to 20.

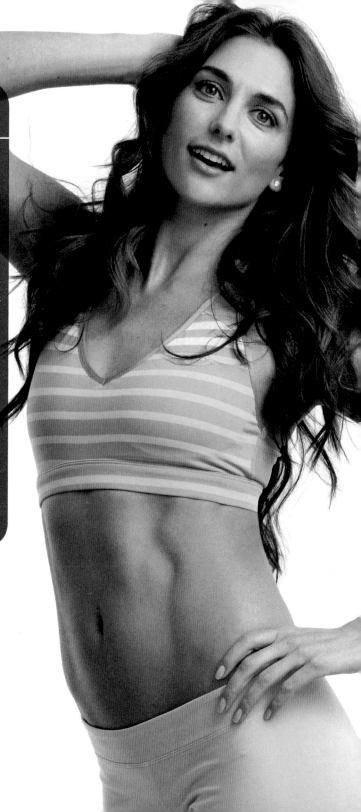

CHAPTER
**04**

# Reshape Your Body in Record Time

## The easiest fat-loss plan ever!

**A**forgiving and flexible fitness mentality—doing any amount of exercise wherever and however possible—can be a productive and effective way to drop pounds. This book is packed with routines that give you plenty of options, based on your schedule, your mood, and what type of equipment you have (or don't have). Translation: There is no excuse to skip a workout. Ever.

But while freestyling your way through weekly workouts may offer variety, it can also make it harder to develop a consistent routine—especially for beginners. Without a set plan, a daily commitment to hit the gym can quickly slide. For many women, the problem is finding a program they can get into.

 **SHAPE-UP** SETBACK

The biggest mistake that people make when performing this style of workout is that they don't rest enough, says dos Remedios. "The key is to select a work period that lets you go hard for the entire duration, then making sure it's paired with an adequate (mandatory) rest period that allows you to recharge your batteries so you can go hard again on the next round."

"The key to creating a maintainable fitness training plan is to address both our strength and cardio needs in short, simple, and effective workouts," says Robert dos Remedios, CSCS, strength and conditioning director at the College of the Canyons in Santa Clarita, California. He knows a thing or two about that winning combination—he, quite literally, wrote the book (*Cardio Strength Training*) on it. The two workouts you'll find in this chapter blend functional, balanced strength training in a circuit with short rest breaks to boost the cardiovascular benefits without compromising all-important lean muscle mass (which helps you burn even more calories after your workout). Oh yeah, and while many programs take about 45 minutes (sometimes more), you'll be done and on your way in 24 minutes.

Here's how to do it: Complete three routines each week on nonconsecutive days, alternating between Workout A and Workout B (so A-B-A during the first week, B-A-B during the second week, etc.). For each workout, start with the first exercise and complete as many reps as you can in 30 seconds, then rest 30 seconds; repeat this pattern until you've completed each move. That's 1 set. Repeat three more times for a total of 4 sets (it should take you about 20 minutes). If you're a beginner (or it's been longer than 2 months since you've last exercised), repeat just one more time for a total of 2 sets.

Each workout also includes a high-intensity, 4-minute "afterburn finisher" (look for the "Turn It Up" arrow at the end). Think of it like extra credit, and aim to complete this exercise after most workouts— even if you're pretty tired. "It gives you a chance to stamp the exclamation point on a great workout—one more chance to throw an extra log on that metabolic furnace you're trying to ignite," says dos Remedios. It also helps you mentally push past your "limits" and test what your body is capable of achieving.

Best part is, it's just 4 minutes, and it's super simple to complete: Do as many as you can in 20 seconds. Then, rest for 10 seconds. That's 1 set. Do 8 of them.

*"Things do not happen.*
*Things are made to happen."*

—JOHN F. KENNEDY

# WORKOUT A AT A GLANCE

### 1 DUMBBELL SKIER SWING

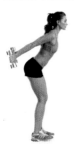

### 2 DUMBBELL GOBLET SQUAT

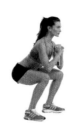

### 3 SUSPENDED PUSHUP

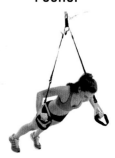

### 4 DUMBBELL ROW

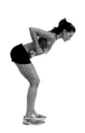

### 5 BODY SAW

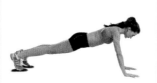

### TURN IT UP!

JUMP ROPE

# WORKOUT A THE EXERCISES

## →1 DUMBBELL SKIER SWING

Hold a pair of dumbbells and stand with
your feet hip-width apart. Push your hips
back and bring the weights behind you
(A), then quickly thrust your hips forward
and swing the dumbbells to shoulder
height (B). That's 1 rep; continue in a
fluid, consistent motion.

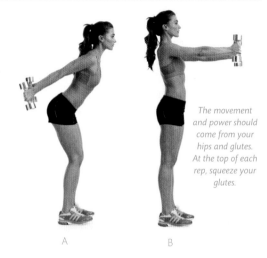

*The movement
and power should
come from your
hips and glutes.
At the top of each
rep, squeeze your
glutes.*

A                              B

## →2 DUMBBELL GOBLET SQUAT

Stand with your feet hip-width apart
and hold a dumbbell vertically in front
of your chest, with both hands cupping
the dumbbell head (A). Push your hips
back and bend your knees to lower into
a squat (B). Push yourself back to start.
That's 1 rep.

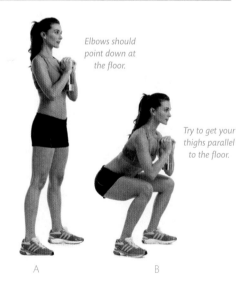

*Elbows should
point down at
the floor.*

*Try to get your
thighs parallel
to the floor.*

A                              B

# WORKOUT A THE EXERCISES

## → 3 SUSPENDED PUSHUP

Secure a TRX or other suspension system, face away from the anchor point with your feet shoulder-width apart, and hold both handles in front of your chest, arms extended (A). Bend your elbows to lower your chest toward the handles (performing a pushup), keeping a straight line from head to heels (B). Pause, then press back to the starting position. That's 1 rep.

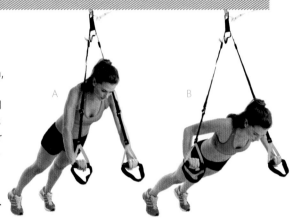

A

B

### SIMPLE ▶ SWAP

Don't have access to a suspension system like TRX? Do this elevated pushup instead.

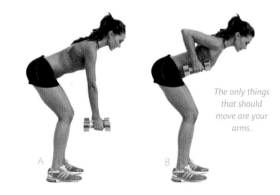

*Place hands slightly wider than shoulder width.*

*Lower your body in a straight line.*

## → 4 DUMBBELL ROW

Holding a pair of dumbbells, stand with your feet hip-width apart, knees bent, arms hanging straight, palms facing each other; bend forward to lower your torso toward the floor (A). Pull your shoulder blades together and row the weights toward your chest (B). Return to the start. That's 1 rep.

*The only things that should move are your arms.*

A

B

# WORKOUT A THE EXERCISES

## → 5 BODY SAW

Place your feet on Valslides and get into a pushup position, hands under your shoulders (A). Keeping your body in a straight line from head to heels, push your feet away from you as far as you can (B). Pull back to start, pressing through your palms. That's 1 rep.

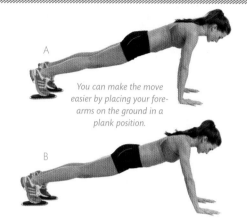

A

*You can make the move easier by placing your fore- arms on the ground in a plank position.*

B

---

**SIMPLE ▷ SWAP**   You can also use small towels or even paper plates in place of the Valslides.

---

**TURN IT UP!**

## JUMP ROPE

Grab the handles of a jump rope, starting with the rope behind you. Keeping your body upright and elbows close, make small circles with your wrists to swing the rope over your head. Jump off the floor as the rope passes your feet, and land softly on the balls of your feet. Continue as quickly as possible.

# WORKOUT B AT A GLANCE

## 1 JUMP SQUAT

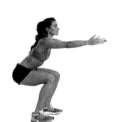

## 2 WALKING LUNGE

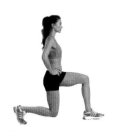

## 3 DUMBBELL PUSH PRESS

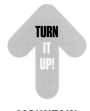

## 4 SUSPENDED ROW

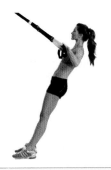

## 5 ALTERNATING BAND ROTATIONS

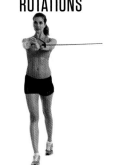

**TURN IT UP!**

## MOUNTAIN CLIMBER

### ➜ 1 JUMP SQUAT

Standing with your feet hip-width apart, sit your hips back to lower into a squat, raising your arms in front of you at shoulder height (A). Press through your heels to jump as high as you can off the ground, swinging your arms behind you (B). That's 1 rep. Land softly and immediately lower into your next squat.

*Keep your chest up and core tight.*

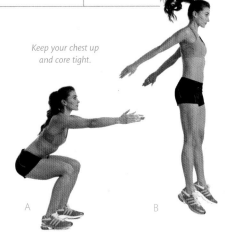

A            B

# WORKOUT B THE EXERCISES

## → 2 WALKING LUNGE

Stand with your feet hip-width apart, hands on your hips (A). Step forward with your left leg and lower your body until both knees are bent 90 degrees (B). Press through your left heel and bring your right foot forward as you return to standing. That's 1 rep. Repeat on the other side and continue alternating.

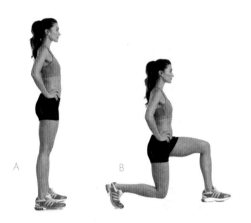

A          B

## → 3 DUMBBELL PUSH PRESS

Hold a pair of dumbbells at shoulder height, palms facing each other, feet hip-width apart. Bend your knees slightly (A), then stand and press the dumbbells overhead, straightening your arms completely (B). That's 1 rep.

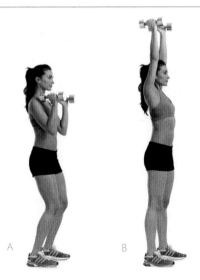

A          B

## → 4 SUSPENDED ROW

Secure a TRX or other suspension system and face the anchor point, holding both handles in front of your chest, arms straight, feet shoulder-width apart (A). Keep your shoulders back; bend your elbows to pull your body toward the anchor point (B). Pause, then slowly return to start. That's 1 rep.

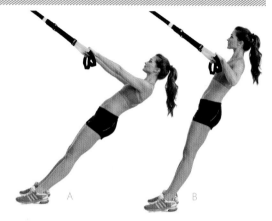

A          B

*You can adjust the level of difficulty of this move by where you place your feet. As you walk your feet farther away from you, you will be pulling a higher percentage of your own body weight.*

## SIMPLE ▶ SWAP

Don't have access to a suspension system like TRX? Do this inverted row instead. *Quick tip:* The higher it is, the easier the exercise will be.

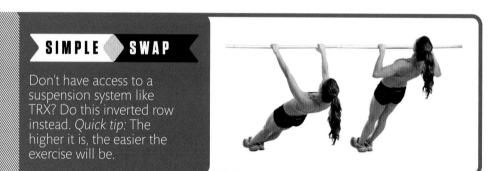

# WORKOUT B THE EXERCISES

## → 5 ALTERNATING BAND ROTATIONS

Stand facing a resistance band (secured a few feet away from you at chest height) and grab the handle with both hands, then step away until you feel tension (A). Brace your core and pull the handle to the right while rotating your hips and shoulders (B). Pause, then return to start. That's 1 rep. Repeat on the left side and continue alternating.

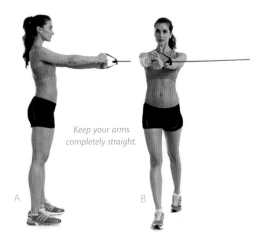

*Keep your arms completely straight.*

A                                              B

## TURN IT UP!

## MOUNTAIN CLIMBER

Start at the top of a pushup position, with your body forming a straight line from head to heels. Keeping your abs braced and back flat, pick up your right foot and bend your knee toward your chest. Return to start then repeat with the other foot; continue alternating. (Refer to the photo on page 67)

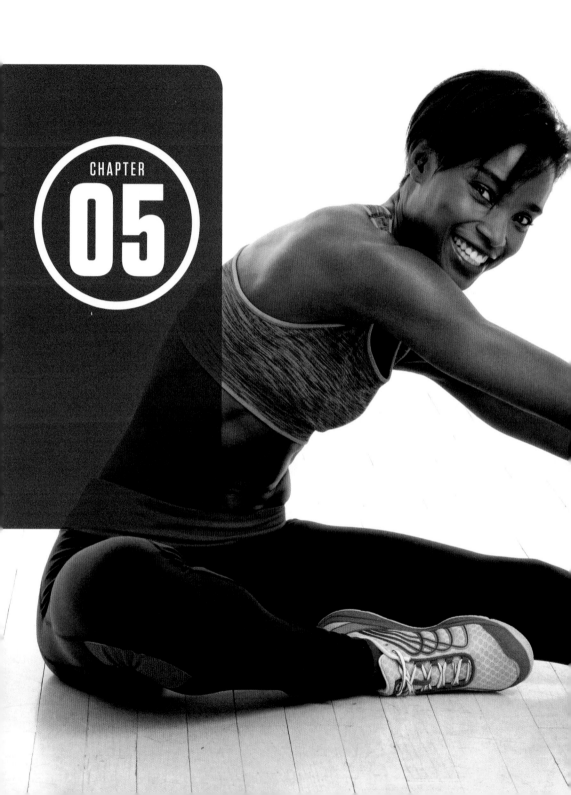

CHAPTER

**05**

# 5-Minute Fat Blasters

*Turbocharge your metabolism and get lean fast*

**H**ere's the thing about the relationship between time and exercise: Even if everyone could find 5 free minutes each day (and I'll safely assume most can), the majority of us wouldn't use that time to work out.

Why? For starters, most women assume that it's not enough time to achieve anything significant. (Which, I should point out, I'm not altogether arguing with.) Then, there's the fact that not many workout programs are created for super-short time frames. So what ends up happening is, the ambitious few with a something-is-better-than-nothing attitude do a few minutes of crunches, pushups, and lunges in their living room while they watch TV. Better than nothing? Sure, I guess. Best they can do? Not even close.

# Maximize Every Minute

▶ The workouts in this chapter are designed specifically for those days when you're short on time—or unmotivated, or tired, or can't make it to the gym. Five exercises, 5 minutes. That's all it takes to rev up your metabolism and build lean muscle.

Just like sprints on a treadmill or in spin class, you have to push hard and fast the entire time. That's what helps dial up the calorie burn and leaves a lingering impression on your metabolism. But while plenty of exercises can leave your lungs burning and muscles aching in the same amount of time, these moves—like the ones by dos Remedios in the previous chapter—are designed based on an intentional selection of movement patterns that, when paired together, give you an effective and balanced total-body workout. (I like to call them POM-style workouts, which stands for "purpose of movement.") Not only will they build strength and work your major muscle groups, but the workouts in this chapter also help develop rotational strength, core stability, hip mobility, and overall flexibility. Translation: In as little as 5 minutes, these workouts will help you build functional, balanced strength—and, of course, kick-start your fat burners.

Intentionally minimal—you won't need anything more than dumbbells (I recommend having at least two pairs, one heavier and one lighter) and a box, bench, or step—these workouts are adaptable to your needs. They can be used as a filler workout in between sessions of your regular strength program. (When your schedule is just too hectic, committing to 5 minutes is an efficient and effective way to maintain consistency.) And when you're not pressed for time, you can repeat the same workout three to five times for a full-length circuit workout. (They make great back-pocket workouts, for when you get to the gym with no plan and need something effective and easy to remember.) Or mix and match a few of the workouts for a longer session that has a wider variety of moves.

## INTERVAL EXCHANGE

Pick one of these two intervals to complete any of the following workouts. Both burn calories, build muscle, and blast fat, but each generates a slightly different metabolic response. Switching between them not only helps speed up results, it also offers just enough variety to fight mental fatigue.

### ⟶ 30:30

Complete as many reps as you can in 30 seconds, then rest for 30 seconds before moving on to the next exercise. (Rest 60 seconds at the end if you're doing more than one round.) Choose the heaviest weights that allow you to work for the entire time and maintain proper form, but challenge you to complete the set.

### ⟶ 50:10

Complete as many reps as you can in 50 seconds, then rest for 10 seconds before moving on to the next exercise. (Rest 60 seconds at the end if you're doing more than one round.) You'll need to use lighter weights, but because you'll be able to perform more reps, it should still be tough to finish a set.

# WORKOUT 1 AT A GLANCE

### 1 STEP UP WITH KNEE DRIVE (LEFT)

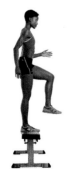

### 2 STEP UP WITH KNEE DRIVE (RIGHT)

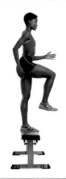

### 3 ALTERNATING BENT-OVER ROW

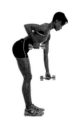

### 4 PUSHUP

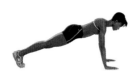

### 5 DUMBBELL SQUAT AND OVERHEAD PRESS

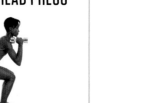

# WORKOUT 1 THE EXERCISES

## →1 STEP UP WITH KNEE DRIVE (LEFT)

Stand in front of a step or bench and place your left foot on top of it (A). Push down through your left heel, pressing your body straight up onto the bench while driving your right knee up (B). Reverse the movement to return to the start. That's 1 rep.

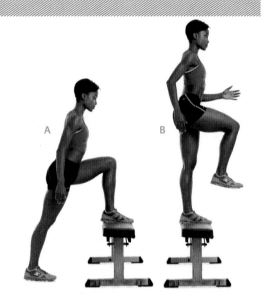

## →2 STEP UP WITH KNEE DRIVE (RIGHT)

Repeat this exercise using the opposite leg.

## →3 ALTERNATING BENT-OVER ROW

Hold a pair of dumbbells and stand with your feet hip-width apart. Bend forward at the hips to lower your torso toward the floor, letting the dumbbells hang at arm's length directly from your shoulders (A). Without raising or rotating your torso, pull the right dumbbell toward your chest (B); pause, then lower your right arm (that's 1 rep) while rowing the left weight toward your chest. Continue alternating.

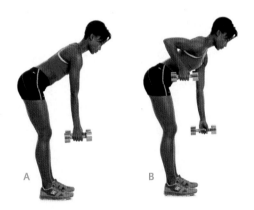

*Alternating places a greater demand on your core and lower back to stabilize your body. To make the move easier, raise and lower both weights together.*

## → 4 PUSHUP

Place your hands shoulder-width apart on the floor and extend your legs behind you (A). Lower your body until your chest nearly touches the floor (B). Pause, then push back to start as quickly as possible. That's 1 rep.

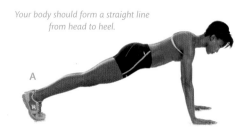

*Your body should form a straight line from head to heel.*

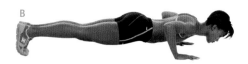

## → 5 DUMBBELL SQUAT AND OVERHEAD PRESS

Hold a pair of dumbbells at shoulder height and stand with your feet hip-width apart, then sit your hips back and lower into a squat (A). Push through your heels to stand, pressing the dumbbells over-head (B). Lower the weights to the start-ing position. That's 1 rep.

*Keep your chest up and core tight as you squat.*

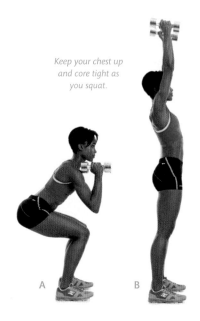

# WORKOUT 2 AT A GLANCE

### 1 MARCHING GLUTE BRIDGE

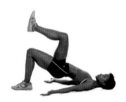

### 2 INVERTED SHOULDER PRESS

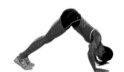

### 3 ALTERNATING SWITCH LUNGE

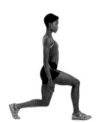

### 4 SKATER HOPS

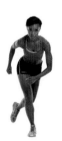

### 5 ROTATING T EXTENSION

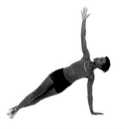

## →1 MARCHING GLUTE BRIDGE

Lie on your back with your knees bent, feet flat on the floor. Rest your arms on the floor, palms up. Raise your hips so your body forms a straight line from shoulders to knees (A). Brace your abs and lift your right knee toward your chest (B). Hold for 2 seconds, then lower your right foot. Repeat with the other leg. That's 1 rep.

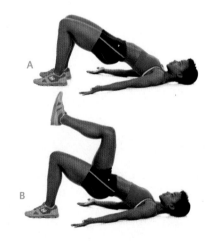

A

B

# WORKOUT 2 THE EXERCISES

## → 2 INVERTED SHOULDER PRESS

Start in a pushup position, hands slightly
wider than shoulder width, then move
your feet forward and raise your hips so
that your torso is nearly perpendicular
to the floor (A). From that position, bend
your elbows to lower your body until
your head nearly touches the floor (B).
Pause, push back to start. That's 1 rep.

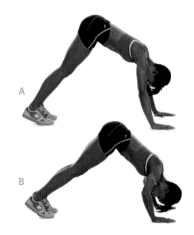

A

B

**SIMPLE SWAP**

Place your feet on
a step or bench
to increase the
challenge.

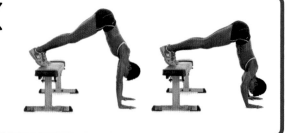

## → 3 ALTERNATING SWITCH LUNGE

Step your right leg forward and bend
both knees to lower into a lunge (A).
Press through your right heel to return to
standing, keeping your foot lifted, then
immediately step your right foot back
and lower into a lunge (B). Press through
your left heel to return to standing. That's
1 rep.

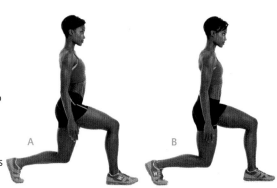

A

B

# WORKOUT 2 THE EXERCISES

## → 4 SKATER HOPS

Stand on your left foot with your left
knee slightly bent and your right foot
slightly off the floor (A). Jump to the right
and land on your right foot, bringing
your left foot (B). That's 1 rep. Jump to the
left and continue alternating as quickly as
possible.

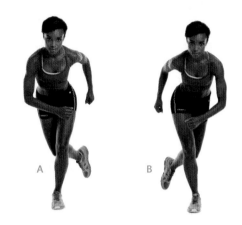

## → 5 ROTATING T EXTENSION

Start in a pushup position (A). Keeping
your arms straight and your core engaged, shift your weight onto your left
arm, rotate your torso to the right, and
raise your right arm toward the ceiling so
that your body forms a *T* (B). Hold for
3 seconds, then return to start and repeat
on the other side. That's 1 rep.

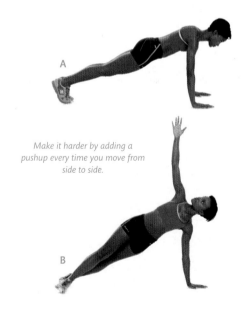

*Make it harder by adding a
pushup every time you move from
side to side.*

# WORKOUT 3 AT A GLANCE

### 1 DUMBBELL SPLIT JERK

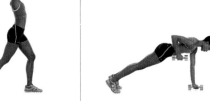

### 2 PUSHUP-POSITION ROW

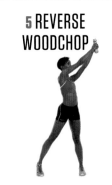

### 3 ALTERNATING LATERAL LUNGE

### 4 REVERSE WOODCHOP

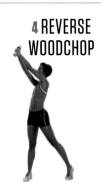

### 5 REVERSE WOODCHOP

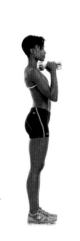

## →1 DUMBBELL SPLIT JERK

Hold a pair of dumbbells at shoulder height, palms facing each other, feet hip-width apart (A). Dip your knees, then quickly press the dumbbells directly overhead as you jump your legs apart so that you land in a staggered stance, one foot in front of the other (B). Step or jump back to start, lowering the weights back to your shoulders. That's 1 rep.

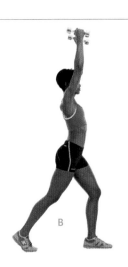

A   B

# WORKOUT 3 THE EXERCISES

## → 2 PUSHUP-POSITION ROW

Get into a pushup position with your hands resting on dumbbells, feet slightly more than hip-width apart (A). Pull one weight toward the side of your chest (B). Lower and repeat on the other side. That's 1 rep.

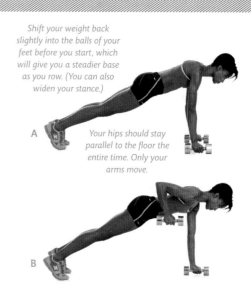

*Shift your weight back slightly into the balls of your feet before you start, which will give you a steadier base as you row. (You can also widen your stance.)*

A

*Your hips should stay parallel to the floor the entire time. Only your arms move.*

B

## → 3 ALTERNATING LATERAL LUNGE

Holding a pair of dumbbells at your sides (A), step to the left and bend your right knee to lower into a side lunge. Lower the dumbbells toward your right foot (B). Press through your right heel to return to start. That's 1 rep. Repeat on the other side and continue alternating.

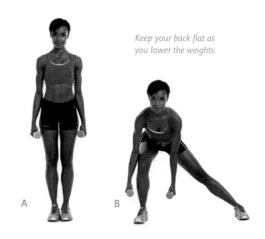

*Keep your back flat as you lower the weights.*

A

B

### 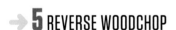 4 REVERSE WOODCHOP

Grab a dumbbell with both hands and stand with your feet wider than hip width, bend your knees, and lower the weight to the side of your left thigh (A). In one motion, press through your heels to stand, and raise the weight over your right shoulder, arms straight and core tight (B). Reverse the movement to return to start. That's 1 rep.

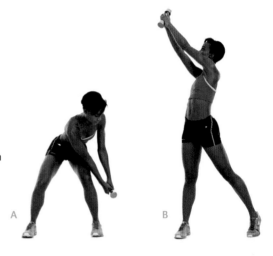

A

B

### 5 REVERSE WOODCHOP

Repeat the above exercise, this time starting with the weight outside your right thigh, and raising it over your left shoulder.

*"The way to get started is to quit talking and begin doing."*

—WALT DISNEY

# WORKOUT 4 AT A GLANCE

### 1 STRAIGHT-LEG DUMBBELL DEADLIFT

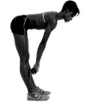

### 2 OVERHEAD DUMBBELL SPLIT SQUAT (RIGHT LEG)

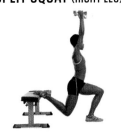

### 3 OVERHEAD DUMBBELL SPLIT SQUAT (LEFT LEG)

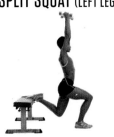

### 4 SIDE-TO-SIDE JUMPS

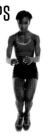

### 5 CROSS-BODY MOUNTAIN CLIMBER

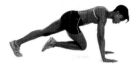
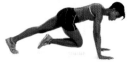

## ➡ 1 STRAIGHT-LEG DUMBBELL DEADLIFT

Hold a pair of dumbbells in front of your thighs, feet hip-width apart (A). Push your hips back and hinge forward to lower your torso until it's almost parallel to the floor, keeping the weights close to your body (B). Return to standing, still keeping the weights close to your body (as if you're shaving your legs with the dumbbells). That's 1 rep.

*Squeeze your glutes and push your hips forward as you stand. Your hips should initiate the movement, not your chest, to avoid relying on your lower back.*

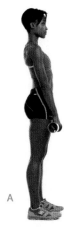
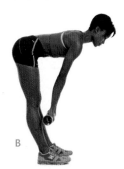

A

B

# WORKOUT 4 THE EXERCISES

## → 2 OVERHEAD DUMBBELL SPLIT SQUAT (RIGHT LEG)

Grab a pair of dumbbells and stand about 2 feet in front of a step or bench; bend your left knee to place the top of your foot on it and raise the weights overhead, arms straight and core tight (A). Bend your knees to lower your body toward the ground (B). Push through your right heel to stand. That's 1 rep.

## → 3 OVERHEAD DUMBBELL SPLIT SQUAT (LEFT LEG)

Repeat the above exercise, starting with your right foot on the bench.

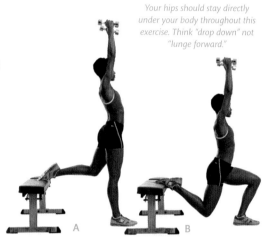

*Your hips should stay directly under your body throughout this exercise. Think "drop down" not "lunge forward."*

A          B

*Holding the weights overhead increases the demand on your core. If your form starts to falter at any time, bend your elbows to bring the weights to shoulder height, or lower your arms to your sides and continue.*

## → 4 SIDE-TO-SIDE JUMPS

Stand with your arms at your sides, feet together (A). Jump to the left with both feet together (imagine you're jumping over a 5-inch cone) (B), landing softly on the balls of your feet; that's 1 rep. Immediately jump to the right, and continue going back and forth as quickly as possible.

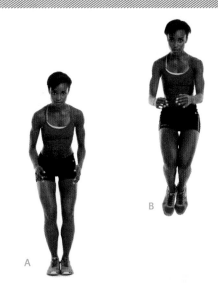

## → 5 CROSS-BODY MOUNTAIN CLIMBER

Start in a pushup position, core and glutes engaged (A). Keeping your back flat and hips level, bend your right knee toward your left shoulder (B). Return to the start and repeat with your left leg. That's 1 rep.

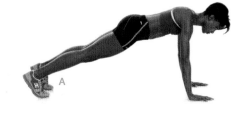

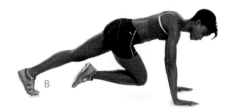

# WORKOUT 5 AT A GLANCE

| | | |
|---|---|---|
| **1 BENT-KNEE DEADLIFT** <br> 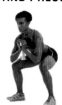 | **2 SINGLE-ARM ROTATIONAL ROW** <br> (RIGHT ARM) <br> 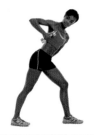 | **3 SINGLE-ARM ROTATIONAL ROW** <br> (LEFT ARM) <br> 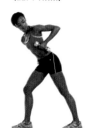 |
| **4 GOBLET SQUAT WITH ROTATION AND PRESS** <br>  | **5 PLANK DUMBBELL DRAG** <br> 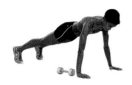 | |

# WORKOUT 5 THE EXERCISES

## →1 BENT-KNEE DEADLIFT

Set a pair of dumbbells on the floor in front of you. Keeping your chest lifted, sit back and bend your knees to squat down and grab the dumbbells with an over-hand grip (A). Press through your heels to stand, squeezing your glutes and pushing your hips forward (B). Slowly lower the dumbbells to the floor. That's 1 rep.

*Don't pull the weights with your arms (which can stress your lower back). Instead, think "push" with your hips.*

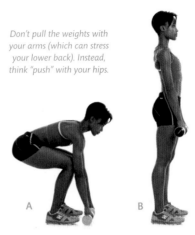

## →2 SINGLE-ARM ROTATIONAL ROW (RIGHT ARM)

Stand with your left foot about 2 feet in front of your right, holding a dumbbell in your right hand, palm facing your body. Bend your knees and hinge forward to lower your torso toward the floor, the weight hanging straight from your shoulder (A). Brace your core and pull the dumbbell toward the right side of your chest, rotating your torso to the right (B). Pause, then lower back to start. That's 1 rep.

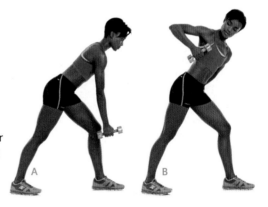

## →3 SINGLE-ARM ROTATIONAL ROW (LEFT ARM)

Repeat the same exercise, this time with the weight in your left hand and your right foot in front of your left.

## →4 GOBLET SQUAT WITH ROTATION AND PRESS

Stand with your feet about hip-width apart and hold a dumbbell vertically in front of your chest, with both hands cupping the dumbbell head (A). Bend your knees and push your hips back to lower your body until your thighs are parallel to the ground. In one motion, stand up and rotate your feet and torso to the left as you press the weight over your left shoulder (B). Reverse the movement to return to start and repeat to the other side. That's 1 rep. Continue alternating.

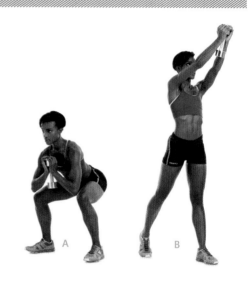

## →5 PLANK DUMBBELL DRAG

Place a dumbbell on the floor and get into a pushup position, feet slightly wider than hip-width, weight outside your left hand (A). Keeping your core tight and hips parallel to the floor, reach your right hand under your body, grab the weight, and pull it to the right (B). Place your right hand back on the floor (C). That's 1 rep. Reach your left arm over and continue alternating.

*The weight of the dumbbell increases the difficulty of this move. If you're unable to maintain proper form (keeping your hips parallel to the floor, body in a straight line), use a lighter dumbbell. You can also complete this as a bodyweight exercise (simply reaching underneath your body to the other side) to build core stability before adding a dumbbell.*

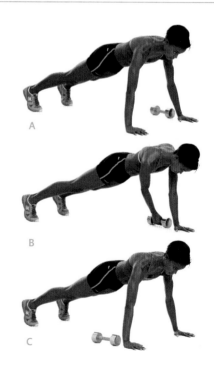

# WORKOUT 6 AT A GLANCE

## 1 SUMO SQUAT WITH LATERAL RAISE

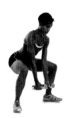

## 2 DUMBBELL CHEST PRESS

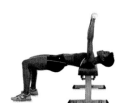

## 3 PLANK WALKUP

## 4 DUMBBELL LUNGE WITH ROTATION

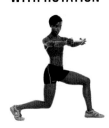

## 5 LOW-BOX LATERAL SHUFFLE

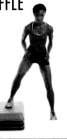

## ➜ 1 SUMO SQUAT WITH LATERAL RAISE

Grab a pair of dumbbells and stand with your feet wider than shoulder-width apart, toes turned out. Sit your hips back and bend your knees to lower into a squat, arms straight and dumbbells between your knees, palms facing each other (A). In one motion, press through your heels to stand and raise both dumbbells to shoulder height (B). Slowly reverse the movement and immediately lower into another rep.

*Focus on being explosive as you stand and raise the weights, but controlled and steady as you lower them.*

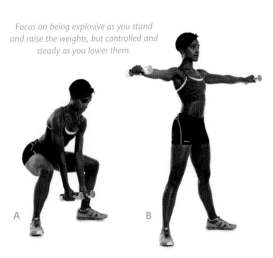

A

B

## → 2 DUMBBELL CHEST PRESS

Grab a pair of dumbbells and position your upper back on a bench with your knees bent, feet flat on the floor; raise your hips to form a straight line from shoulders to knees, and press the dumbbells over your chest, arms straight and palms facing away from you (A). Lower your arms until the weights are even with your chest (B). Press back to the starting position. That's 1 rep.

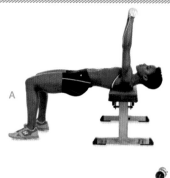

A

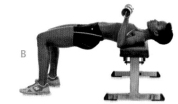

B

*This variation recruits more of your glutes, hamstrings, and core throughout the exercise. You can make it easier by lying completely on the bench; you can make it harder by swapping the bench for a stability ball. But don't forget the goal of this exercise: to challenge your chest and arms. So choose a variation that allows you to lift a challenging weight with proper form.*

## → 3 PLANK WALKUP

Position your forearms on the ground, elbows directly under your shoulders, and extend your legs behind you (A). Place your right hand flat on the floor (B), and then your left hand, straightening your arms to press your body into a pushup position (C). Reverse the movement, lowering onto your right forearm and then your left, to return to the start. That's 1 rep. Repeat, leading with your left hand, and continue alternating.

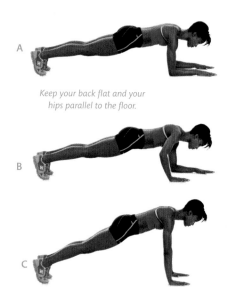

A

*Keep your back flat and your hips parallel to the floor.*

B

C

# WORKOUT 6 THE EXERCISES

## → 4 DUMBBELL LUNGE WITH ROTATION

Grab a dumbbell with both hands and raise it to shoulder height in front of you, arms straight and feet hip-width apart (A). Keeping your core tight and your chest up, step forward with your left foot and lower your body until your front thigh is nearly parallel to the floor, rotating your shoulders and torso to the right (B). Rotate back to the center as you press through your right heel to return to the standing position. That's 1 rep. Repeat on the other side and continue alternating.

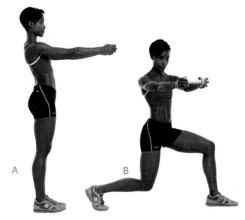

A    B

*If at any point during this exercise it's too difficult to keep your arms straight out in front of you, bend your elbows to bring the weight close to your chest and continue the move as directed. If that is too challenging, ditch the dumbbell and complete the remaining reps of your set as a bodyweight exercise.*

## → 5 LOW-BOX LATERAL SHUFFLE

Stand to the right of a low box or step and place your left foot on it; bend your knees slightly and keep your chest up (A). Push off your left foot and jump over the box to your left, landing with your right foot on the box and your left foot on the floor, knees bent (B). Quickly return to start. That's 1 rep.

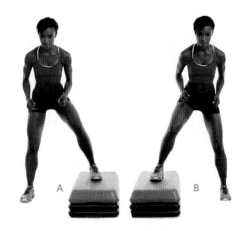

A    B

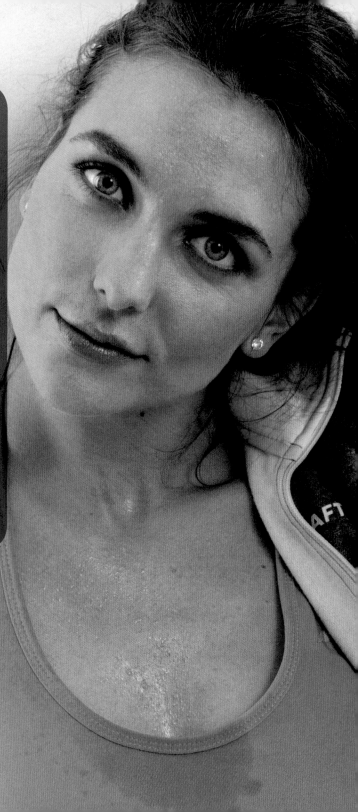

# Simple Workouts, Serious Results

*Slim down faster—with less equipment*

There's a lot of fitness equipment out there. It's all over infomercials, your gym, maybe even your home. And there are some terrific tools to help make you stronger, faster, and leaner, while creating more dynamic, fun, and effective workouts. With the right combination, you can amplify your body's innate ability to build muscle and burn fat—and see even more impressive results.

But sometimes even with a dream team of equipment, the sum of their individual genius doesn't add up to an unmatched workout. In fact, when you need a stability ball, step, kettlebell, cable machine, and resistance band—all for one 20-minute workout—the time it takes to set up from one piece of equipment to the next can lower the overall intensity (or perhaps worse, tack on precious minutes to your total gym time).

The innovative routines in this chapter are created by some of the top trainers in the country, and each is scientifically designed to give you the most effective workout in under 30 minutes—using only one piece of equipment (or none!). It's all about simplicity—dialing back the extras in your sweat session so you can make the most out of every rep, every set, every minute. And without fumbling from one piece of equipment to the next—or worse, waiting to work out during rush hour at the gym—you'll save time with each workout. So whether you're in a crowded gym or at home with basic equipment, there's a routine that will work for you.

# Total-Body Training

▶ Ask 20 trainers and exercise physiologists what the single best exercise is, and you'd probably hear nearly 20 different answers. But, without doubt, one that would make the list is the burpee. It's on the short list of best fat-burning, bodyweight exercises of all time, thanks to how many major muscle groups it activates in a single rep. Not to mention, because you're moving quickly up and down off the ground, it can generate a significant cardiovascular response in as little as 60 seconds. (Don't believe me? Take the "1-Minute Burpee Challenge!" on page 144.) It's no surprise why this one-move wonder is used in gyms, boot camps, and on CrossFit boxes across the country.

Here's the problem: Improper form can easily destroy the burpee's effectiveness. Many people lack the mobility in their hips, ankles, and upper back to do the standard version properly, says BJ Gaddour, CSCS, CEO of StreamFIT.com. These problems are only intensified as people quickly get tired and sloppy. Rather than stop and rest, they're often encouraged to continue flopping around like fish out of water, all for the sake of getting those few extra reps in. It may *feel* like you're working hard, but in reality you're just increasing your risk of injury.

The number of reps you complete isn't the only way to change the intensity of the burpee. I recruited BJ to help me create a Burpee Spectrum (see pages 140–143), which ranks 10 variations from hardest to easiest so you can find the burpee that fits your fitness level. You can also use it to safely adjust any workout: Rather than cranking out reps with sloppy form, scale back by choosing an easier variation and continue working.

# THE BURPEE SPECTRUM

**HARDEST**

10
SINGLE-ARM

9
SINGLE-LEG

8
WITH PUSHUP
AND JUMP

7
WITH PUSHUP

6
WITH JUMP

5
CLASSIC

4
BOX WITH PUSH-
UP AND JUMP

3
BOX WITH
PUSHUP

2
BOX WITH
JUMP

1
BOX STEP-OUT

**EASIEST**

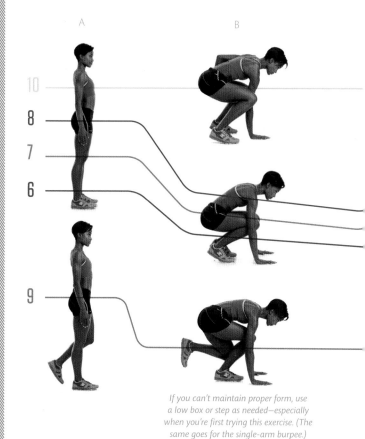

A     B

10

8

7

6

9

*If you can't maintain proper form, use a low box or step as needed—especially when you're first trying this exercise. (The same goes for the single-arm burpee.)*

## 10 SINGLE-ARM BURPEE

Stand with your feet about shoulder-width apart (A). Sit your hips back and lower into a squat, placing one hand in front of you on the floor in the center of your body (B). Jump both feet back into a pushup position (C); quickly reverse the movement to return to the start (D,E). Repeat with the other arm; continue alternating.

## 9 SINGLE-LEG BURPEE

Stand on one foot (A). Keeping one foot off the ground, squat down as far as you can, and place your hands on the floor (B). Jump back into a pushup position, keeping your one foot elevated (C). Reverse the movement to return to start (D,E). Repeat on the other leg; continue alternating.

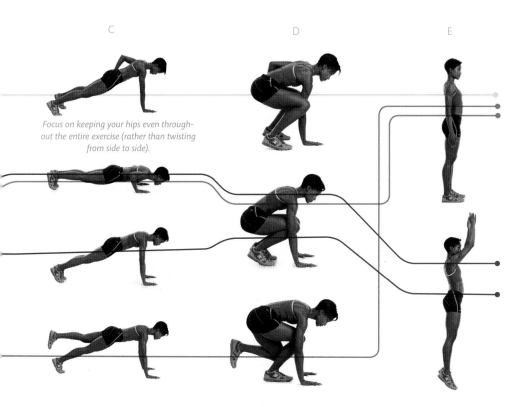

C       D      E

*Focus on keeping your hips even throughout the entire exercise (rather than twisting from side to side).*

## 8 BURPEE WITH PUSHUP AND JUMP

Stand with your feet about shoulder-width apart, arms at your sides (A). Push your hips back, and squat down to place your hands on the floor (B). Jump back into a pushup position, then bend your elbows to lower your body toward the floor (C); quickly reverse the movement (D), then jump up into the air (E).

## 7 BURPEE WITH PUSHUP

Stand with your feet about shoulder-width apart, arms at your sides (A). Push your hips back and squat down to place your hands on the floor (B). Jump both feet back into a pushup position, then bend your elbows to lower your body toward the floor (C); quickly reverse the movement (D) to return to start (E).

## 6 BURPEE WITH JUMP

Stand with your feet about shoulder-width apart, arms at your sides (A). Push your hips back, and squat down to place your hands on the floor (B). Jump both feet back into a pushup position (C); quickly reverse the movement (D) and immediately jump up into the air (E).

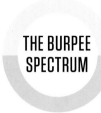

# THE BURPEE SPECTRUM

## HARDEST

**10**
SINGLE-ARM

**9**
SINGLE-LEG

**8**
WITH PUSHUP
AND JUMP

**7**
WITH PUSHUP

**6**
WITH JUMP

**5**
CLASSIC

**4**
BOX WITH PUSH-
UP AND JUMP

**3**
BOX WITH
PUSHUP

**2**
BOX WITH
JUMP

**1**
BOX STEP-OUT

## EASIEST

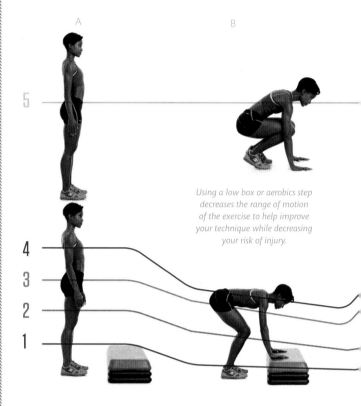

A        B

5

4

3

2

1

*Using a low box or aerobics step decreases the range of motion of the exercise to help improve your technique while decreasing your risk of injury.*

## 5 CLASSIC BURPEE

Stand with your feet about shoulder-width apart, arms at your sides (A). Push your hips back, and squat down to place your hands on the floor (B). Kick your legs back into a pushup position (C); quickly reverse the movement to return to standing (D,E).

## 4 BOX BURPEE WITH PUSHUP AND JUMP

Stand with your feet about shoulder-width apart, arms at your sides (A). Push your hips back, and squat down to place your hands on the box or step (B). Jump both feet back into a pushup position, then bend your elbows to lower your chest toward the box (C); reverse the movement (D), and immediately jump up into the air (E).

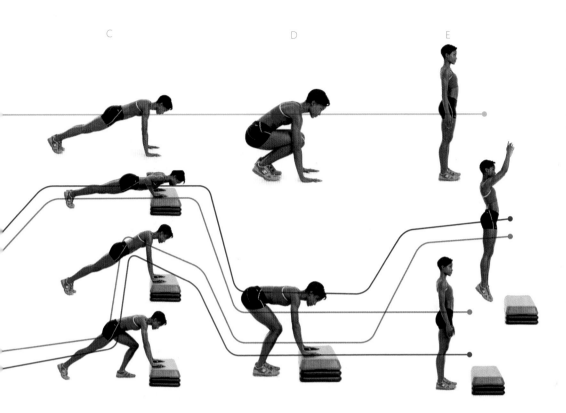

### 3 BOX BURPEE WITH PUSHUP

Stand with your feet about shoulder-width apart, arms at your sides (A). Push your hips back, and squat down to place your hands on the box or step (B). Jump both feet back into a pushup position, then bend your elbows to lower your chest toward the box (C); quickly reverse the movement to return to standing (D,E).

### 2 BOX BURPEE WITH JUMP

Stand with your feet about shoulder-width apart, arms at your sides (A). Push your hips back, and squat down to place your hands on the box or step (B). Jump both feet back into a pushup position (C); quickly reverse the movement (D), and immediately jump up into the air (E).

### 1 BOX STEP-OUT BURPEE

Stand with your feet about shoulder-width apart, arms at your sides (A). Push your hips back, and squat down to place your hands on the box or step (B). Step your feet back one at a time into a pushup position (C); pause, then reverse the movement to return to standing (D,E).

## THE ONE-MOVE WORKOUT

The burpee is so efficient that it can actually be used as a complete, total-body workout. Torch fat, burn calories, and build muscle in a single move with this simple program from Gaddour.

Select a burpee from the spectrum, and start at Level 1. Complete 6 reps per minute, using the remaining time in each minute to rest. Repeat for up to 15 minutes. Once you can complete all 15 minutes, move on to Level 2 using the same burpee variation. When you've worked up to completing Level 3 for the entire 15 minutes, return to Level 1 and choose the next (more difficult) variation on the Burpee Spectrum.

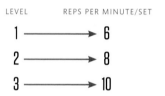

| LEVEL | REPS PER MINUTE/SET |
|---|---|
| 1 | 6 |
| 2 | 8 |
| 3 | 10 |

*You may think that doing the same move over and over would become ineffective. But because the volume of your workout increases as you move up the levels, you'll ensure your body never adapts to the single exercise.*

## 1-MINUTE BURPEE CHALLENGE!

Select a burpee from the spectrum and do as many reps as you can in 60 seconds. If you notice your form starting to slide, scale down to an easier variation, so you can keep scoring benefits—without upping your risk of injury. On the flip side, as your fitness increases and the set starts to feel easy, move up to the next level.

"*What progress,
you ask,
have I made?
I have begun to be
a friend to myself.*"

—HECATO

# The Greatest Bodyweight Workout Ever

➡ You don't need a gym membership to sculpt a great body. In fact, you don't even need equipment. Think about the classic pullup—for many women, it's freakin' hard to do, and yet there are no weights involved. That's because when you do a pullup, your body is in a position that forces your back and arms to lift your entire body weight, so the scientific laws of motion and leverage are working against you. In other words, physics turns your body into an uber-efficient resistance machine.

Problem is, just like with any exercise routine, over time your body adapts and basic bodyweight exercises—like squats, pushups, and, yes, even pullups—become easier. Increasing the number of reps can offset the plateau, but only to an extent.

This workout, created by Mark Verstegen, world-renowned athletic performance specialist and founder of Athletes' Performance in Phoenix, has three distinct phases that increase in difficulty so you can keep seeing results. During each phase, you'll move quickly through four compound sets; like their cousin the superset, compound sets are an incredible time-saver because they transition from one move to the next with no downtime. Unlike supersets, which work two opposing muscle groups back to back, compound sets work the *same* muscle group. (Take the first two moves for example: a bodyweight squat followed immediately by an isometric wall squat.) This back-to-back pattern helps recruit even more muscle fibers and creates greater strength gains—all without adding external resistance (think: dumbbells).

Here's how to do it: Start with Workout 1. Refer to the directions for Phase 1 in the chart on page 147 and complete the prescribed number of reps for A1 and A2, moving from one to the next without rest; move on to B1 and B2 and repeat, and continue until you've finished all of the exercises. A full round of all four compound sets is considered one circuit. Rest up to 60 to 90 seconds, then repeat for two to four total circuits.

There are three ways to make this workout more difficult (read: to keep seeing progress and avoid hitting plateaus): First, you can increase the volume by moving through the three phases using the same workout. (So the exercises stay the same, but the reps and duration increase.) Or you can also increase the exercise difficulty by going from Workout 1, to Workout 2, to Workout 3 (but keeping the phase the same). Lastly, you can change both factors—volume and exercise difficulty—at the same time: Start in Phase 1 with Workout 1, then move to Phase 2 with Workout 2, and finally Phase 3 with Workout 3. The choice is yours!

| PHASE | PHASE | PHASE |
|:---:|:---:|:---:|
| 1 | 2 | 3 |
| A1 B1 C1 | A1 B1 C1 | A1 B1 C1 |
| **10 REPS** | **15 REPS** | **20 REPS** |
| A2 B2 C2 D1 D2 | A2 B2 C2 D1 D2 | A2 B2 C2 D1 D2 |
| **30 seconds** | **40 seconds** | **60 seconds** |
| (or 15 each side) | (or 20 each side) | (or 30 each side) |

# WORKOUT 1

## → A1 BODYWEIGHT SQUAT

Stand with your feet slightly wider than
hip-width apart, and raise your arms
straight in front of you at shoulder height
(A). Keeping your arms straight and your
chest lifted, sit your hips back and bend
your knees to lower your body until
your thighs are parallel to the ground (B).
Pause, then press through your heels to
return to standing. That's 1 rep.

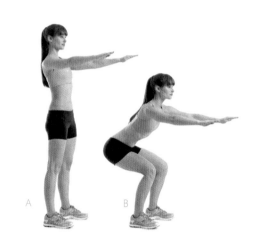

A                    B

## → A2 ISOMETRIC WALL SQUAT

Stand with your back against a wall, your
feet about 2 feet in front of you, hip-
width apart. Bend your knees to lower
your body until your knees are bent at
90 degrees. Hold.

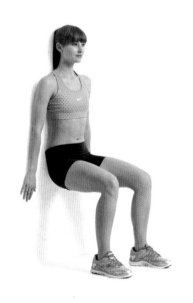

# WORKOUT 1

## → B1 MODIFIED WIDE-GRIP PUSHUP

Start in a pushup position with your hands wider than shoulder-width apart on the floor, then place your knees on the ground, so your body forms a straight line from shoulders to knees (A). Bend your elbows to lower your body toward the floor in a straight line (B). Press back up to the start. That's 1 rep.

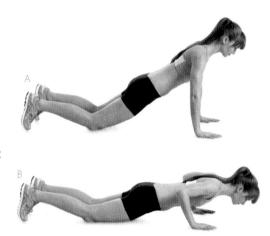

## → B2 NARROW-GRIP MODIFIED ISOMETRIC PUSHUP

Start in a pushup position with your hands closer than shoulder-width apart on the floor, then place your knees on the ground, so your body forms a straight line from shoulders to knees. Bend your elbows to lower your body until your elbows form 90-degree angles. Hold.

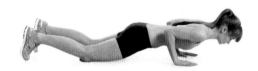

*Keep your shoulders safe by imagining that you're trying to push the ceiling up with your back, without moving your arms.*

## → **C1** SPLIT SQUAT

Stand with your legs staggered, your right foot about 2 feet in front of your left (A). Bend your knees to lower your body until your right thigh is parallel and your shin is perpendicular to the floor (B). Straighten your legs to return to the start. That's 1 rep. Complete all reps on that leg, then switch sides and repeat.

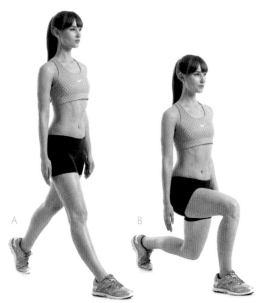

A       B

## → **C2** GLUTE BRIDGE

Lie faceup on the floor with your knees bent, feet flat on the floor, and your arms to your sides, palms facing up. Press through your heels and raise your hips off the ground so your body forms a straight line from shoulders to knees. Hold.

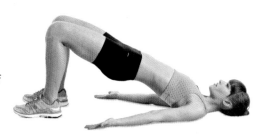

# WORKOUT 1

## → D1 PLANK

Place your forearms on the ground with your elbows directly under your shoulders, and extend your legs so that your body forms a straight line from head to heels. Brace your core and hold.

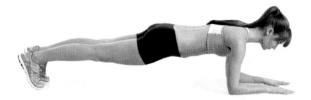

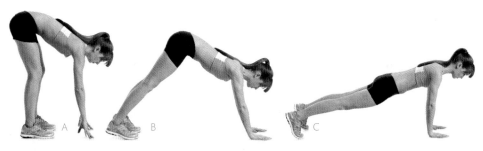

A    B    C

## → D2 INCHWORM

Stand with your feet hip-width apart, bend over, and touch the floor in front of your feet with both hands (A). Keeping your legs straight and core tight, walk your hands forward as far as you can without letting your hips drop (B,C). Pause, then slowly walk your feet toward your hands. That's 1 rep.

*Take tiny steps with your hands and feet. The baby steps torch your hamstrings and calves, while your arms and shoulders are constantly at work. And the farther your feet get from your hands, the harder your core has to work to keep you stable.*

# WORKOUT 2

### → A1 ALTERNATING LATERAL LUNGE

Stand with your feet hip-width apart, arms raised to shoulder height (A). Keeping your arms raised and your chest lifted, step out to the left with your left leg; bend your knee and sit back to lower into a side lunge, keeping your back flat (B). Press through your right heel to return to standing. That's 1 rep; repeat on the other side and continue alternating.

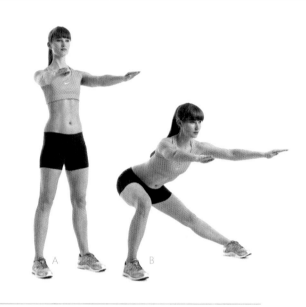

### → A2 ALTERNATING SINGLE-LEG ISOMETRIC WALL SQUAT

Stand with your back against a wall, your feet about 2 feet in front of you, hip-width apart. Bend your knees to lower your body until your knees are bent at 90 degrees (A). Extend your right leg out in front of you, shin parallel to the floor (B). Hold for 1 or 2 seconds, then switch sides and repeat. Continue alternating.

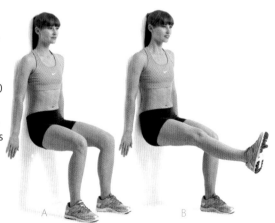

# WORKOUT 2

## → **B1** WIDE-GRIP PUSHUP

Place your hands on the floor wider than shoulder-width apart, and extend your feet behind you into a pushup position, so your body forms a straight line from head to heels (A). Bend your elbows to lower your body toward the floor in a straight line (B). Press back up to the start. That's 1 rep.

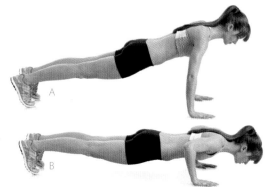

## → **B2** NARROW-GRIP ISOMETRIC PUSHUP

Place your hands on the floor closer than shoulder-width apart, and extend your feet behind you into a pushup position, so your body forms a straight line from head to heels. Keeping your core tight, bend your elbows to lower your body in a straight line until your elbows form 90-degree angles. Hold.

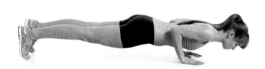

# WORKOUT 2

## → C1 ALTERNATING REVERSE LUNGE

Stand with your feet hip-width apart, arms at your sides (A). Step back with your left leg and lower your body until your right knee is bent at 90 degrees (B). Push back up to the start. That's 1 rep. Complete all reps on that leg, then switch sides and repeat.

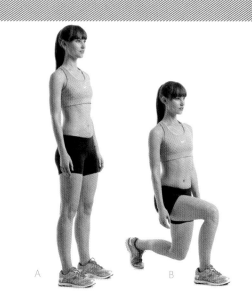

## → C2 MARCHING GLUTE BRIDGE

Lie faceup on the floor with your knees bent, feet flat on the floor, and your arms to your sides, palms facing up. Press through your heels and raise your hips off the ground so your body forms a straight line from shoulders to knees (A). From this position, raise your right foot off the ground, knee bent at 90 degrees, until your shin is parallel to the floor (B). Hold for 2 or 3 seconds, then lower your right foot and repeat with the left foot. Continue alternating.

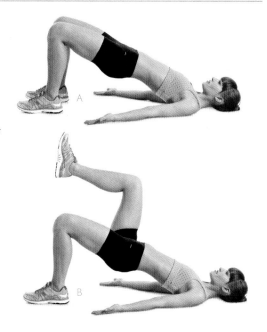

# WORKOUT 2

## → D1 SIDE PLANK

Lie on your left side and place your forearm on the ground with your elbow directly under your shoulder, your legs straight and stacked. Lift your hips so your body forms a straight line from head to heels. Hold, then switch sides and repeat.

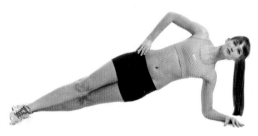

## → D2 INCHWORM WITH PUSHUP

Stand with your feet hip-width apart, bend over, and touch the floor in front of your feet with both hands (A). Keeping your legs straight and core tight, walk your hands forward until they are directly under your shoulders, and your body forms a straight line from head to heels (B). Bend your elbows to lower your chest to the ground (C), then straighten your arms; slowly walk your feet toward your hands. That's 1 rep.

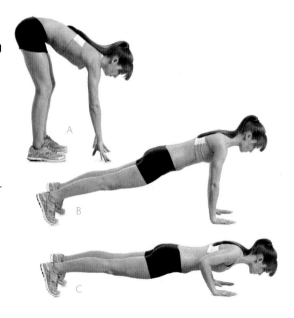

# WORKOUT 3

## → **A1** SINGLE-LEG BODYWEIGHT SQUAT

Stand with your feet hip-width apart, arms raised to shoulder height (A), and raise your left foot off the ground. Keeping your arms raised and your chest lifted, sit your hips back and bend your right knee to lower your body as far as you can, keeping your left leg extended off the ground in front of you (B). Press through your heel to return to standing. That's 1 rep. Complete all reps on that leg, then switch sides and repeat.

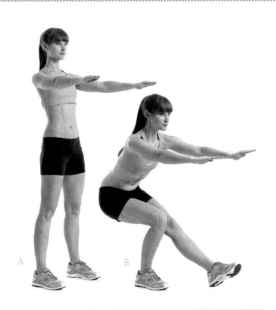

A                    B

## → **A2** SINGLE-LEG ISOMETRIC WALL SQUAT

Stand with your back against a wall, your feet about 2 feet in front of you, hip-width apart. Bend your knees to lower your body until your knees are bent at 90 degrees. Extend your right leg out in front of you, shin parallel to the floor. Hold for 1 or 2 seconds, then switch sides and repeat. Continue alternating.

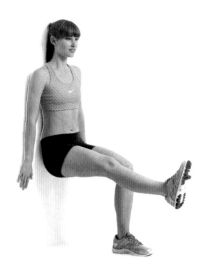

# WORKOUT 3

### ➡ **B1** ALTERNATING SINGLE-LEG WIDE-GRIP PUSHUP

Place your hands on the floor wider than shoulder-width apart, and extend your feet behind you into a pushup position, so your body forms a straight line from head to heels. Raise your left leg (A), then bend your elbows to lower your body toward the floor in a straight line (B). Press back up to the start and lower your leg. That's 1 rep. Repeat on the other side and continue alternating.

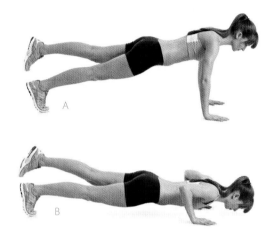

### ➡ **B2** SINGLE-LEG NARROW-GRIP ISOMETRIC PUSHUP

Place your hands on the floor closer than shoulder-width apart, and extend your feet behind you into a pushup position, so your body forms a straight line from head to heels. Raise your left leg, then bend your elbows to lower your body in a straight line until your elbows form 90-degree angles. Hold.

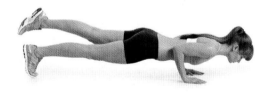

## → **C1** REAR-FOOT ELEVATED SPLIT SQUAT

Stand about 2 feet in front of a step or bench and place the top of your left foot on it (A). Bend your knees to lower into a lunge until your left knee grazes the floor, keeping your chest upright and hips directly under your body (B). Push through your right heel to stand. That's 1 rep. Complete all reps with that leg, then switch sides and repeat.

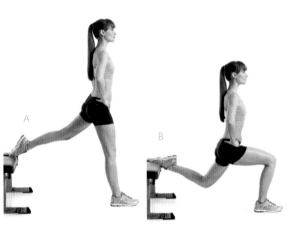

## → **C2** SINGLE-LEG HIP EXTENSION

Lie faceup on the floor with your left knee bent and your right leg straight (A). Raise your right leg until it's in line with your left thigh. Push your hips upward, keeping your right leg elevated, until your body forms a straight line from shoulders to right ankle (B). Pause, then slowly lower your body and leg back to the start. That's 1 rep. Complete all the reps with that leg, then switch sides and repeat.

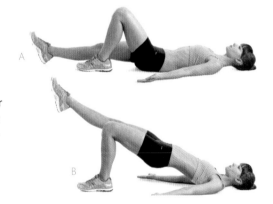

# WORKOUT 3

## ➡ **D1** ROLLING PLANK

Start in the plank position, with your forearms on the ground and your legs extended behind you (A). Rotate your torso to the side, rolling onto your left forearm and stacking your right foot on top of your left in a left-side plank (B). Pause, then return to the start, and repeat on the other side.

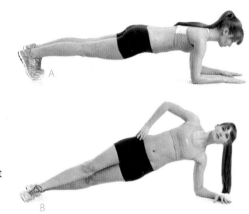

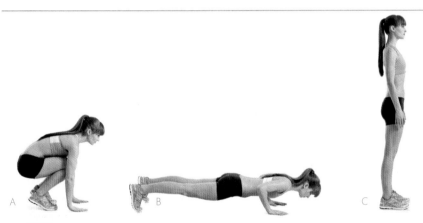

## ➡ **D2** BURPEE

Stand with your feet slightly wider than shoulder-width apart, arms at your sides. Push your hips back, bend your knees, and lower your body into a squat and place both hands on the floor in front of you (A). Jump both feet back into a pushup position (B); bring your feet back into a low squat and quickly jump up into the air, swinging your arms overhead then moving back to standing position (C). That's 1 rep.

# 5 Laws of Bodyweight Workouts

Good news: All bodyweight exercises can be just as challenging (and effective) as a pullup. You just have to know how to tailor them to your fitness level—and then adapt them when that level changes.

## LAW #1: TO GET LEANER, BE LONGER

**THE SCIENCE:** As you increase the distance between the point of force (your target muscles) and the end of the object you're trying to lift (your body), you decrease your mechanical advantage. Translation: The longer your body, the weaker you become and the more your muscles have to work. This is the major difference between "girly" pushups and regular ones. When you get off your knees your core muscles have to work a whole lot harder to support more of your body weight.

**APPLY IT:** Raise your hands above your head so your arms are straight and in line with your body during lunges, squats, crunches, and situps. Too hard? Split the distance by putting your hands behind your head.

## LAW #2: TAKE THE SPRING OUT OF YOUR STEP

**THE SCIENCE:** When you lower your body during any exercise, your muscles build up what's known as elastic energy. It works like a coiled spring: The elasticity allows you to bounce back to the starting position and reduces the amount of work your muscles have to do.

**APPLY IT:** Take a 4-second pause at the bottom position of any exercise. That's how long it takes to discharge all the elastic energy of a muscle. Without the bounce, you'll force your body to recruit more muscle fibers to get you moving again.

## LAW #3: GO THE DISTANCE

**THE SCIENCE:** Physics defines work as force (here, that's how much you weigh) times distance. Since you can't increase force beyond your own body weight without an external load (like a dumbbell), the only way to work more is to move farther during each rep.

**APPLY IT:** For bodyweight exercises—such as lunges, pushups, and sit-ups—your range of motion ends at the floor. The solution: Move the floor farther away. Try placing your front or back foot on a step when doing lunges, or position your hands or feet on a step when doing pushups.

## LAW #4: ADD A TWIST

**THE SCIENCE:** Human movement happens on three geometric planes: the sagittal plane (front-back and up-down), the frontal plane (side to side), and the transverse plane (rotation). Many common bodyweight exercises—like squats and side lunges—are performed on the first two planes. But we rarely train our bodies on the transverse plane, despite using it all the time in our everyday lives: when walking, for example.

**APPLY IT:** Simply rotate your torso to the right or left in exercises such as lunges, situps, and pushups; you'll fully engage your core in addition to the muscles those moves are intended to target.

## LAW #5: GET OFF THE FLOOR

**THE SCIENCE:** The less of an object's surface area (in this case, your body) that touches a solid base (the floor), the less stable that object is. Fortunately, we have a built-in stabilization system: our muscles. So knocking yourself a little off kilter makes you exercise harder and enlists more muscles.

**APPLY IT:** Hold one foot in the air during pushups, squats, and planks.

# Tone Every Inch

⬤ Looking to shake up your normal routine? Sculpt every muscle in your body with a suspension system like TRX, which creates resistance from two things always at your disposal: body weight and gravity. And it does so at a fraction of the cost of a personal trainer or gym membership.

This portable, affordable tool is a favorite of fitness experts like renowned performance trainer Todd Durkin, CSCS, owner of Fitness Quest 10 and author of *The Impact! Body Plan*. And it's not just reserved for his all-star athletes like Drew Brees; he uses this tool with all of his clients. That's because it's simple yet versatile, allowing Durkin to choose from hundreds of functional exercises to build strength, endurance, core stability, and mobility at any fitness level. (You can simply change the way you position your body to increase or decrease the intensity.) Plus, the suspension trainer forces your core to work harder during every exercise, accelerating your flat-belly goals.

Build a stronger, leaner body from head to toe and burn fat fast with this workout created by Durkin. Starting with Circuit 1, complete the prescribed number of reps for each exercise, moving from one to the next without resting. Repeat for a total of three sets, then rest 2 minutes. Follow the same pattern to complete three sets of Circuit 2, then continue to Circuit 3 and perform two sets.

# CIRCUIT 1

### → 1 SUSPENDED SQUAT JUMPS

Grab the TRX handles in both hands and stand facing the anchor point with your arms extended, feet shoulder-width apart (A). Sit your hips back and bend your knees to lower your body until your thighs are parallel to the ground. Keeping your arms straight, press through your heels and quickly jump up as high as you can with both feet off the ground (B). Land softly and immediately lower into another rep. Do 10.

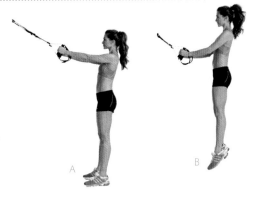

### → 2 SUSPENDED CHEST PRESS

Stand facing away from the anchor point, feet hip-width apart, and hold the handles in front of you with arms extended at shoulder height, palms facing the floor (A). Walk your feet away from you and lean forward so your body forms a straight line from head to heels. Keeping your core tight, bend your elbows to lower your chest toward the handles (B). Pause, then press back to the start. That's 1 rep. Do 10.

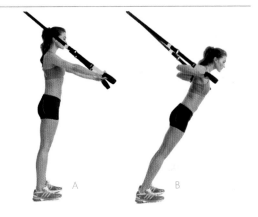

### → 3 SUSPENDED ROW

Grab the TRX handles in both hands and stand facing the anchor point with feet shoulder-width apart and arms straight in front of you. Lean back and walk your feet forward to the appropriate resistance angle (A). Keeping your shoulders pulled down and back, bend your elbows to pull your chest toward the handles (B). Pause, then return to the start with a slow, controlled movement. That's 1 rep. Do 10.

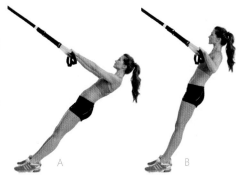

# CIRCUIT 2

## ➡ 1 SUSPENDED BICEPS CURLS

Grab the TRX handles in both hands with an underhand grip, and stand facing the anchor point with feet shoulder-width apart and arms straight in front of you. Lean back and walk your feet forward to the appropriate resistance angle (A). Keeping your shoulders down and your body in a straight line, bend your elbows to curl the handles toward your shoulders (B). Pause, then return to the start with a slow, controlled movement. That's 1 rep. Do 10.

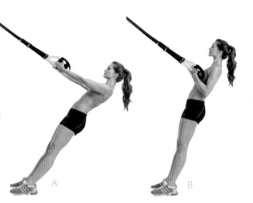

## ➡ 2 SUSPENDED OVERHEAD TRICEPS EXTENSIONS

Stand facing away from the anchor point, feet hip-width apart, and hold the handles with your palms facing down and your arms extended (A). Pressing your body weight into the handles, bend your elbows and lower your body until your hands are behind your head (B). Drive your hands forward and extend your arms to return to the start. That's 1 rep. Do 10.

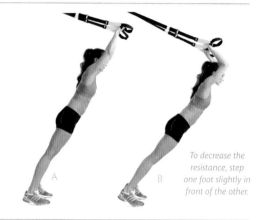

*To decrease the resistance, step one foot slightly in front of the other.*

## ➡ 3 SUSPENDED POWER PULL

Stand facing the anchor point, feet hip-width apart, and hold one handle in your right hand, arm extended at shoulder height. Lean back and walk your feet forward to the appropriate resistance angle (A). Keeping your core tight and your body in a straight line, bend your right elbow to pull your chest toward the handle (B). Pause, then return to the start. That's 1 rep. Do 8, then switch sides and repeat.

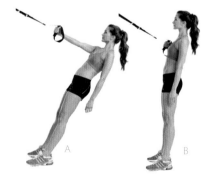

# CIRCUIT 3

## → 1 BURPEE

Stand with your feet about shoulder-width apart (A), then push your hips back and squat down to place your hands on the floor (B). Jump your legs back into a pushup position (C); quickly reverse the movement to return to the start. That's 1 rep. Do 10.

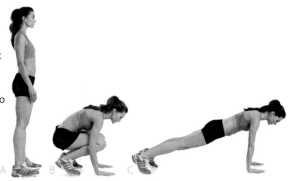

## → 2 SKATER JUMP

Cross your left leg behind your right and lower into a half-squat, your right arm out to the side, left arm across your hips (A). Hop to the left, switching your legs and arms (B). That's 1 rep. Keep hopping quickly from side to side. Do 30.

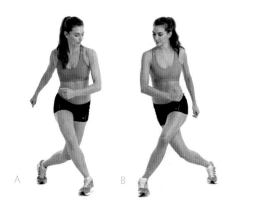

*"It's always too early to quit."*

—NORMAN VINCENT PEALE

# One Dumbbell, One Hot Body

▶ This routine—created by Craig Ballantyne, CSCS, a strength and conditioning coach in Toronto and author of *Turbulence Training*—will incinerate fat and tighten your body in record time. Starting with the first exercise, perform the prescribed number of reps, then rest 30 seconds before continuing to the next move. (You can rest up to a minute, if needed; make it harder by reducing the rest break or dropping it altogether.) Repeat until you've finished the entire circuit, and rest 2 minutes. That's one set; aim to finish as many as you can in the time you have, up to 30 minutes. (Beginners should start with two total.)

## ➜ 1 NARROW-STANCE GOBLET SQUAT

Stand with your feet shoulder-width apart and hold a dumbbell vertically in front of your chest, both hands cupping the dumbbell head (A). Keeping your chest up and your core tight, sit your hips back and squat as low as you can (B). Press through your heels to return to start. That's 1 rep. Do 15.

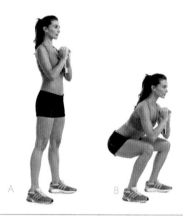

## ➜ 2 SINGLE-ARM BENT-OVER ROW

Place your left knee and left hand on a bench and hold a dumbbell in your right hand at arm's length, palm facing the bench (A). Slowly bend your elbow and pull the dumbbell to your chest (B). Pause, then lower back to the start. That's 1 rep. Do 10, then repeat on the other side.

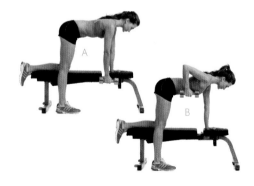

## 3 SINGLE-ARM CHEST PRESS

Lie faceup on a bench, holding a dumbbell in your left hand at chest height (A). Press the weight directly over your shoulder (B). Slowly lower back to start. That's 1 rep. Do 10, then switch arms and repeat.

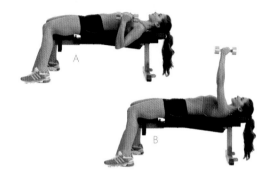

## 4 GOBLET SPLIT SQUAT

Stand with your right foot 2 feet in front of your left and hold a dumbbell vertically in front of your chest (A). Bend your knees to lower your body until your right thigh is parallel to the floor (B). Straighten your legs to return to the start. That's 1 rep. Do 6, then switch legs and repeat.

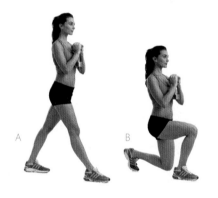

## 5 DUMBBELL SWING

Grab a dumbbell with an overhand grip, feet hip-width apart. Push your hips back, knees slightly bent, and lower your chest to bring the dumbbell between your legs (A). Keeping your core tight, push your hips forward and swing the dumbbell up to shoulder height (B). Reverse the movement, swinging the weight back between your legs. That's 1 rep. Do 15.

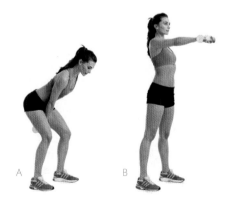

# The Ultimate Kettlebell Workout

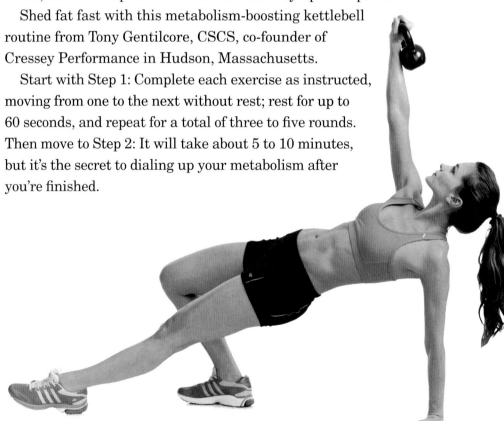

▶ If you think kettlebells are just hyped-up dumbbells, think again. Unlike a dumbbell, a kettlebell's center of gravity shifts during an exercise, increasing the challenge and building coordination. Researchers found that people who did 20-minute kettlebell workouts torched almost 300 calories—and that's just for starters. When you factor in the calories burned after you exercise as your body repairs its muscle fibers, the total expenditure could increase by up to 50 percent.

Shed fat fast with this metabolism-boosting kettlebell routine from Tony Gentilcore, CSCS, co-founder of Cressey Performance in Hudson, Massachusetts.

Start with Step 1: Complete each exercise as instructed, moving from one to the next without rest; rest for up to 60 seconds, and repeat for a total of three to five rounds. Then move to Step 2: It will take about 5 to 10 minutes, but it's the secret to dialing up your metabolism after you're finished.

# STEP 1 AT A GLANCE

**1** KETTLEBELL SUMO DEADLIFT

**2** KETTLEBELL PUSHUP-POSITION ROW

**3** KETTLEBELL REVERSE LUNGE

**4** KETTLEBELL HALO

**5** KETTLEBELL HALF GET-UP

**6** YOGA PUSHUP

STEP 2

SINGLE-ARM FARMER'S WALK SHUTTLE WITH KETTLEBELL SWINGS

## →1 KETTLEBELL SUMO DEADLIFT

Stand with your feet about twice shoulder-width apart and your toes pointed out at an angle. Bend at your hips and knees and grab the kettlebell handle with an overhand grip. Your lower back should be slightly arched, and your arms should be straight (A). Without allowing your lower back to round, pull your torso back and up, thrust your hips forward, and stand up with the kettlebell (B). That's 1 rep. Do 12 to 15.

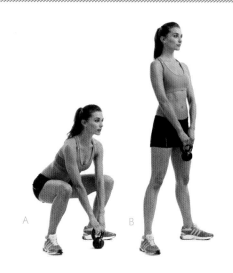

## →2 KETTLEBELL PUSHUP-POSITION ROW

Get in a pushup position with your hand on top of a kettlebell (A). Keeping your hips parallel and back flat, bend your elbow to row the weight toward your chest (B). Pause, then return to start. That's 1 rep. Do 8 to 10, then switch sides and repeat.

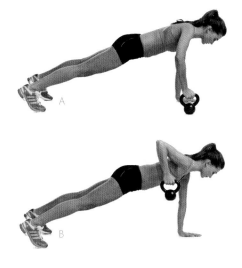

# STEP 1 SCULPT SEXY MUSCLE

### ➔ 3 KETTLEBELL REVERSE LUNGE

Hold the kettlebell handle in your right hand so the bell rests on the back of your forearm (or "racked" position), hand close to your chest and elbow close to your body (A). Brace your core and step back with your right leg and bend both knees to lower your body until both knees form 90-degree angles (B). Pause, then press through your left heel to return to the start. That's 1 rep. Do 10 to 12, then switch sides and repeat.

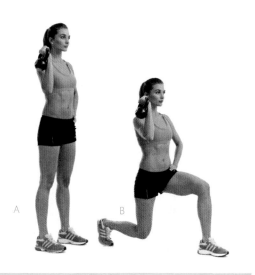

### ➔ 4 KETTLEBELL HALO

Stand with your feet hip-width apart and hold the kettlebell in front of your head, about shoulder height (A). Keeping your core tight and stable, circle the weight counterclockwise around your head (B). That's 1 rep. Do 12 to 15.

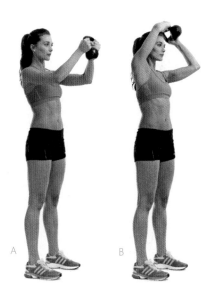

## → 5 KETTLEBELL HALF GET-UP

Lie faceup on the floor with your right knee bent, foot flat on the floor, and your left leg extended straight; hold a kettlebell in your right hand, with your arm directly over your shoulder (A). Roll onto your left forearm and punch the ceiling with your right hand to raise your upper body off the ground (B). Straighten your left arm and place your hand on the floor behind you, so that your upper body forms a *T*; then press into your right heel and raise your hips until they're in line with your knee, raising the weight toward the ceiling (C). Pause, then reverse the movement to return to the starting position. That's 1 rep. Do 8 to 10, then switch sides and repeat.

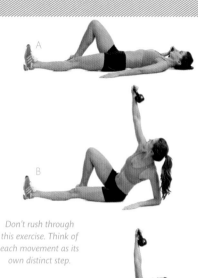
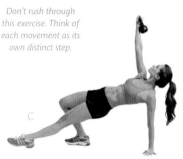
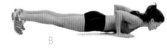

*Don't rush through this exercise. Think of each movement as its own distinct step.*

## → 6 YOGA PUSHUP

Place your hands on the ground directly under your shoulders and extend your legs behind you into a pushup position, with your body forming a straight line from head to heels (A). Bend your elbows to lower your chest toward the ground (B); straighten your arms and as you return to the start, raise your hips up in the air while driving your heels into the ground (downward-facing dog position) (C). Reset to the starting position. That's 1 rep.

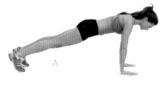
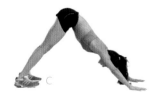

*If that's too difficult, simply remove the pushup and go back and forth from the starting position to downward-facing dog.*

# STEP 2 FIRE UP YOUR FAT BURNERS

## SINGLE-ARM FARMER'S WALK SHUTTLE WITH KETTLEBELL SWINGS

Set up two markers roughly 25 to 30 yards apart. Hold a kettlebell at your right side; walk from one marker to the other, keeping your chest upright (A). Once you reach the other end, position your feet about hip-width apart and hold the kettlebell in front of you with both hands. Push your hips back, slightly bend your knees, and lower your chest to bring the weight between your legs (B). Quickly push your hips forward and swing the weight to chest height (C). Immediately bring the weight between your legs. That's 1 rep. Do 10. Hold the kettlebell in your left hand and walk back to the first marker. Perform another 10 swings. That's one round. Rest 30 to 60 seconds. Repeat for a total of two to four rounds.

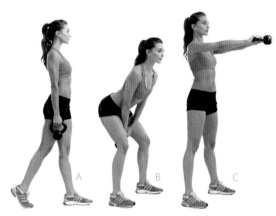

 **SLIM-DOWN SECRET**

Here's a simple way to make the workouts more difficult (and more time-efficient): Lower your rest break at the end of each circuit. So the first week you do it, rest 60 seconds. During the second week, lower it to 50 seconds; for the third week, drop it to 40 seconds, and so on.

# Step Up Your Results

📣 Crank up your calorie burn and score a fierce physique with this explosive 15-minute workout created by David Jack, director of Teamworks Fitness in Acton, Massachusetts. It takes advantage of a traditional cardio step to strengthen your cardiovascular system and tone your muscles at the same time—the ultimate one-two punch for igniting your fat-burning engine. The innovative dynamic exercises Jack uses help boost agility and speed, and because they aren't likely in your everyday routine, you'll stay more focused on the movements. (You *might* even have some fun.)

Using a traditional aerobics step (or a 4- to 6-inch low box), perform the following circuit as instructed below. The key is to move quickly while always maintaining proper form; challenge yourself to squeeze out an extra rep each time you complete this routine.

## ➡ 1 ALTERNATING ELEVATED REVERSE LUNGE

Stand on a step or box (A), then step your left leg onto the floor behind you; bend both knees to lower until your right knee is bent at least 90 degrees (B). Push through the right heel to return to the start. That's 1 rep. Repeat on the other leg and continue alternating for 40 seconds. Rest 20 seconds, then continue to the next exercise.

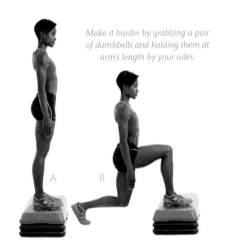

*Make it harder by grabbing a pair of dumbbells and holding them at arm's length by your sides.*

A   B

## → 2 PUSHUP PLANK WALKOVER

Start in a pushup position to the right of a low box or step (A). Place your left hand onto the step (B), then your right (C). Place your left hand on the floor to the left of the step, followed by your right, so that both hands are now on the left side of the step. Reverse to return to the start. That's 1 rep. Continue for 10 seconds, then rest 10 seconds. Repeat three times (1 minute), then move to the next exercise.

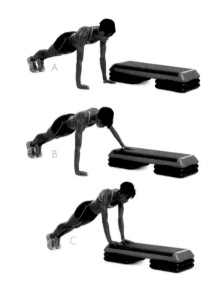

*Make it harder by adding a pushup to the movement on either side of the step or box.*

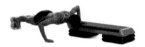

## → 3 SCISSOR SWITCHES

Place the ball of your left foot on the step in front of you (A). Press into the box and jump, switching feet so that your right foot is on the step (B). That's 1 rep. Continue alternating as quickly as possible for 10 seconds, then rest 10 seconds. Repeat three times (1 minute). Rest 20 seconds, then move to the next exercise.

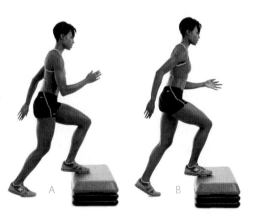

## →4 PLANK WITH ALTERNATING LEG RAISE

Place your forearms on the step, elbows directly under your shoulders, and extend your feet behind you (A). Keeping your core tight and your back flat, raise your right leg off the ground (B). Hold for 3 seconds, then lower and repeat with the other leg. Continue alternating for 30 seconds. Rest 30 seconds, then move to the next exercise.

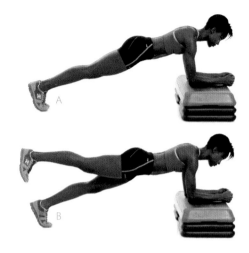

*You only have to raise your foot slightly. Raising too high can throw off your alignment*

## →5 SQUAT AND POP

Place one foot on either side of the step (the narrow portion between your feet); sit your hips back to lower into a half squat, keeping your chest up (A). Quickly jump both feet up onto the box (B), landing softly and immediately jumping to the start, lowering into another squat. That's 1 rep. Continue for 30 seconds, then immediately continue to the next exercise.

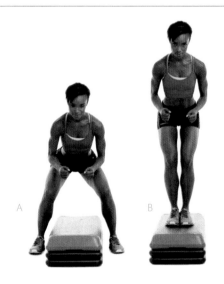

## → 6 SIDE PLANK

Place your left forearm on the step directly under your shoulder; extend your legs and raise your hips so that your body forms a straight line from head to heels. Hold for 20 seconds, then immediately switch sides and repeat. Rest 20 seconds, then continue to the next exercise.

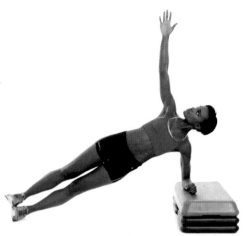

*Focus on squeezing your glutes throughout the movement (it helps strengthen your core, maintain proper alignment, and relieve pressure on your lower back).*

## → 7 THE RUNAROUND

Stand to the side of the step, knees and elbows slightly bent. Quickly step your left foot onto the step (A), followed by your right, and then quickly step off to the other side, your left foot (B) followed by your right. Reverse the movement to return to the starting position. Repeat the lateral step over, then run forward and make a circle around the entire step. That's 1 rep. Immediately repeat the lateral step overs, and continue this pattern for 40 seconds. Rest 40 seconds, then repeat the circuit one more time.

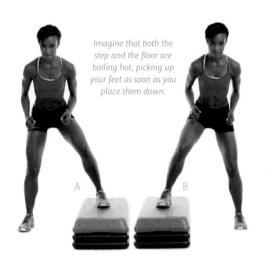

*Imagine that both the step and the floor are boiling hot, picking up your feet as soon as you place them down.*

# The Ball That Does It All

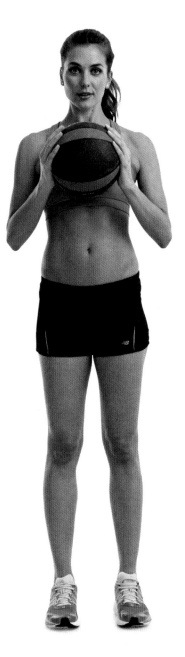

➡ Pop quiz: What piece of fitness equipment can you throw, catch, hold, and lift? The correct answer: a medicine ball. (If you answered "a dumbbell," please don't work out near other people.)

Whether you're throwing it onto the ground or catching it mid-lunge, a medicine ball challenges your core stability and coordination while toning your upper and lower body. This fast-paced circuit workout, created by Hannah Davis, New York City–based personal trainer and co-owner of Gotham Versatile, will blast fat and sculpt muscle in 30 minutes. It's super simple, too: Starting with Circuit 1, complete the prescribed number of reps for each exercise, moving from one to the next without resting. Rest up to a minute (if needed), then repeat two more times for a total of three circuits. Rest 1 to 2 minutes, then continue to Circuit 2 and repeat. Continue this pattern until you've finished the entire workout.

# CIRCUIT 1

## → 1 MEDICINE BALL ROLLING PUSHUP

Get in a pushup position with your right hand on top of a medicine ball and your left hand on the floor, your body in a straight line from head to heels (A). Bend your elbows to lower your chest toward the floor (B), then press back up until your arms are fully extended. Roll the ball to your left, then quickly place your weight on your right hand and place your left hand on top of the ball (C). Do another pushup, then roll the ball back to the start. That's 1 rep. Do 10 to 14.

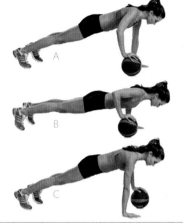

*Make it easier by placing your knees on the ground.*

## → 2 MEDICINE BALL HIP RAISE

Lie faceup on the floor, arms out to your sides with palms up, and place both feet on a medicine ball, knees bent about 90 degrees (A). Squeeze your glutes and raise your hips so that your body forms a straight line from shoulders to knees (B). Pause, then lower back to the start. That's 1 rep. Do 15.

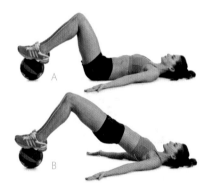

## → 3 MEDICINE BALL TAPS

Place a medicine ball on the ground in front of you and lightly place one foot on top of it, knee bent (A). Keeping your weight over your hips, switch feet so the other foot is on top of the ball (B); continue alternating as quickly as possible, picking your knees up and staying light on the balls of your feet. Do as many taps as you can in 1 minute.

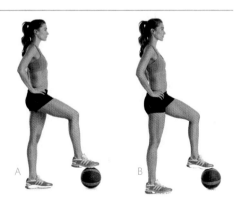

# CIRCUIT 2

## → 1 SQUAT WITH OVERHEAD TOSS

Stand with your feet hip-width apart holding a medicine ball at chest height, elbows bent and close to the body. Sit your hips back and bend your knees to lower your body until your thighs are parallel to the floor (A). Pause, then press through your heels and explosively return to standing as you straighten your arms to press the ball toward the ceiling, releasing it overhead (B). Catch it, bending your knees to absorb the impact. Immediately lower into another rep. Do 15.

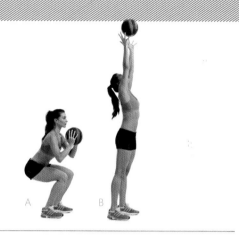

## → 2 MEDICINE BALL DONKEY KICKS

Place the medicine ball on the floor and extend your legs behind you into a pushup position, feet wider than hip-width apart and hands on top of the ball. Keeping your core tight, bend your right knee toward your chest (A), pause, then press your heel up toward the ceiling, knee bent at 90 degrees (B). That's 1 rep. Immediately draw the knee back into the chest and continue for 10 reps, then switch sides and repeat.

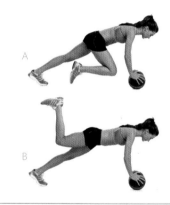

## → 3 BENT-OVER ARM RAISE

Holding a medicine ball with both hands, stand with your feet about shoulder-width apart, knees slightly bent; hinge forward at the hips to lower your torso toward the floor, keeping your back flat, arms hanging straight in line with your shoulders (A). Keeping your arms straight and without changing the position of your torso, brace your core and slowly raise the ball in front of you until your arms are on either side of your head (B). Pause, then slowly lower back to the start. That's 1 rep. Do 12 to 15.

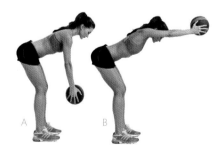

# CIRCUIT 3

## → 1 MEDICINE BALL SEATED TWIST WITH PRESS

Holding a medicine ball, sit on the floor with your knees bent and feet flexed. Keep your back straight and hips facing forward as you twist your torso to the right and touch the weight to the floor next to you (A). Rotate back to the center and press the weight overhead (B), then lower it and rotate to the left (C). Reverse the movement to return to the start. That's 1 rep. Do 10.

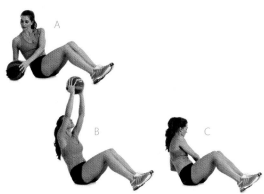

## → 2 MEDICINE BALL BURPEE

Stand with your feet slightly wider than shoulder-width apart, holding a medicine ball at your chest (A). Push your hips back, bend your knees, and squat down to place the ball on the floor with both hands on the ball (B). Kick your legs back into a pushup position (C); quickly reverse the movement to return to standing. That's 1 rep. Do 15.

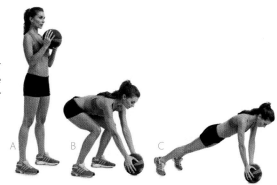

## → 3 AROUND-THE-WORLD LUNGE

Hold a medicine ball in front of your chest, feet shoulder-width apart (A). Take a big step to your left, lowering your body by pushing your hips back and bending your left knee as you circle the ball to the right (B) and bring it over your left foot (C). Press through your left heel to return to the start. That's 1 rep. Repeat on the other side, and continue alternating for a total of 20 reps.

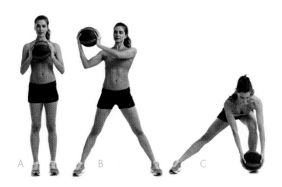

# Sculpt a Knockout Body

▶ Unlike other gym machines that lock you into a fixed movement pattern, the cable machine allows for more functional movements so you can work your muscles from all angles with a greater range of motion. It also keeps your muscles under constant tension, giving you a tough workout, especially your core, which has to work overtime to stabilize your body each time you pull a cable. And it's a one-stop shop: You can get a killer head-to-toe workout without hopping around the gym.

This routine, created by Dan Trink, a strength coach and personal trainer at Peak Performance in New York City, is designed to build lean muscle and amp up your calorie burn during—and after—the workout. Complete 12 to 15 reps of each exercise, moving from one to the next without a break. Rest for 1 minute, then repeat the circuit three more times.

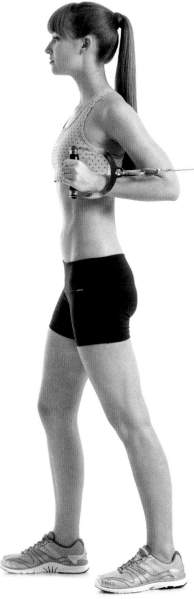

# →1 CABLE SQUAT TO ROW

Grab a universal grips (a strap with two handles) in each hand and stand facing the weight stack, feet hip-width apart. Sit your hips back and bend your knees to lower your body toward the floor (A). As you stand, bend your elbows to row the handles to the sides of your chest (B). That's 1 rep.

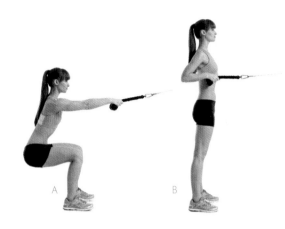

A          B

## SIMPLE ◆ SWAP

Get a similar workout by doing these moves with a resistance band. Choose one with handles and anchor it to a sturdy object (like around a banister or table leg), then perform the exercises as instructed.

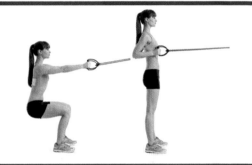

# →2 SINGLE-ARM CABLE CHEST PRESS

Grab a handle (attached at chest height) with your left hand and face away from the machine, elbow bent and palm down. Step your left foot back into a split stance, knees bent (A). Brace your abs and forcefully press the handle forward (B). Do all reps, then switch sides and repeat.

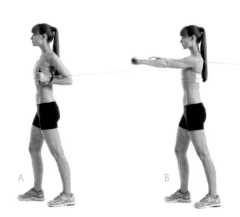

A          B

## 3 CABLE WOODCHOPPER

Secure a handle at the highest point and stand to the right of the machine. Grab the handle with both hands so your arms are extended above your left shoulder, feet wide and knees slightly bent (A). Keeping your arms straight, pull the handle across the front of your body to the outside of your right thigh, shifting your weight from your left foot to your right (B). Slowly return to start. That's 1 rep. Do all reps on that side, then switch sides and repeat.

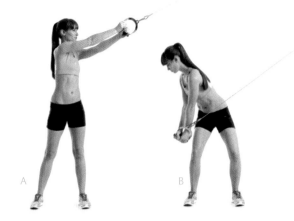

A                    B

## 4 CABLE CORE PRESS

Stand to the right of the cable station and grab the handle (attached at chest height) with both hands at your chest (A). Keeping a tight core, press the handle directly out in front of you (B). Hold for 2 seconds, then return to start. Complete all reps on that side, then turn to face the opposite direction and repeat.

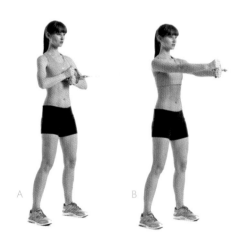

A                    B

# Lean Legs, Flat Abs— Anytime, Anywhere

⯈ Staying fit on the road can be tough, I know. From packing logistics (running shoes take up precious carry-on room) to limited access to equipment or space (like only having access to a weak hotel gym) and just being super busy and tired—it can make fitting in a workout the last thing you want to do.

One of my solutions? Valslides. Created by the amazing Los Angeles–based trainer Valerie Waters, they're an affordable, portable replacement for slide boards that you might find in some gyms. They work on carpet, tile, hardwood floors—pretty much anything other than concrete—to create extra friction during any workout (translation: They make moves more difficult.). And you can throw them in your gym bag, or, if you're like me, your carry-on. (I have taken very few trips without my Valslides.)

This simple routine is one of my go-tos when I need a fast, total-body workout on the road. Complete the prescribed number of reps for each exercise in order, moving from one to the next without rest. Rest for up to a minute, then repeat for a total of two to three circuits.

*"You're one workout away from a good mood."*

—VALERIE WATERS

## →1 VALSLIDE PIKE

Get into a pushup position, hands directly under your shoulders and both feet on a Valslide. Your body should form a straight line from head to heels (A). Keeping your back flat and legs straight, brace your core and raise your hips to pull your feet toward your hands (B). Pause, then slowly return to start. That's 1 rep. Do 12 to 15.

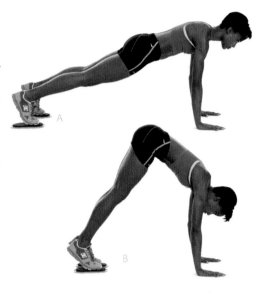

## →2 VALSLIDE CURTSY LUNGE

Place your left foot on a Valslide and stand with your feet hip-width apart (A). In one motion, slide your left foot back and behind your right leg as you bend both knees to lower into a lunge (B). Press through your right heel to return to standing. That's 1 rep. Do 10 to 12, then switch legs and repeat.

*Women often lean forward as they lunge. Focus on moving your leg backward and sitting your hips straight down.*

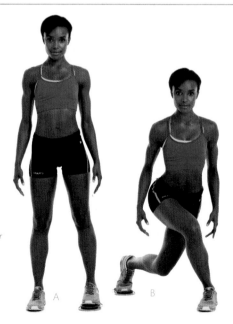

## → 3 VALSLIDE PUSHUP

Place your hands on the floor shoulder-width apart, your right hand on a Valslide, and extend both feet so that you're in a pushup position with your body forming a straight line from head to heels (A). Keeping your core tight, slide your right arm away from your left and bend both elbows to lower your body toward the ground as far as possible (B). Press through your left palm and pull your right hand back to the start. That's 1 rep. Do 6 to 8, then switch hands and repeat.

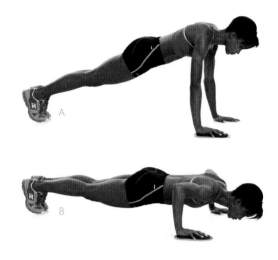

## → 4 SINGLE-LEG VALSLIDE CURL

Lie faceup on the floor with palms up, your left heel on a Valslide, and your right foot flat on the floor, knee bent (A). Squeeze your glutes and raise your hips off the ground. Bend your left knee and pull it toward your butt and in line with your right knee (B). Pause, then reverse the move to return to start. That's 1 rep. Do 6 to 8, then switch legs and repeat

*Make this move more challenging by raising your right foot off the floor and performing the exercise as instructed.*

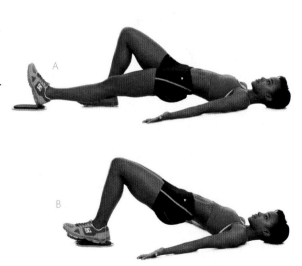

## ➜ **5** VALSLIDE ARM CIRCLE

Place each hand on a Valslide directly under your shoulders and extend your feet behind you into a pushup position, your body forming a straight line from head to heels (A). Keeping your core tight and your hips parallel to the floor, slowly make a large clockwise circle with your right hand (B), returning it under your shoulder. Repeat on the other side. That's 1 rep. Do 15.

*The only part of your body that should move is your arm. Focus on not dropping your shoulders or hips, or twisting side to side. Think "tight as a board" with your core.*

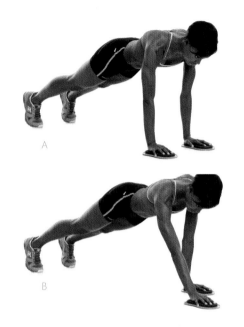

A

B

## ➜ **6** UPSIDE-DOWN SNOW ANGEL

Place your hands on the floor directly under your shoulders; place a Valslide under both feet and extend your legs so that your body forms a straight line from head to heels (A). Without dropping your hips, slide your legs out to the sides as far as you can (B); pause, then slide them back together. That's 1 rep. Do 15.

*Focus on squeezing your glutes and inner thighs with each rep.*

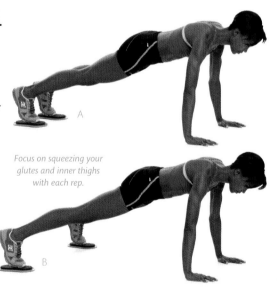

A

B

# Work Out the Kinks

➡ Tend to aching muscles with this foam-roller routine. The moves take about 10 to 15 minutes to complete and hit all your soreness-prone places. Plus, you can do them anytime: during your favorite TV show, before bed, first thing in the morning, or after a workout. Roll over each spot five to 10 times. If a spot feels extra tender, try this: Start below the area, work up to it and hold for a few seconds, then roll through it.

## ➡ 1 CALVES

Sit on the floor with your legs straight out, hands on the floor behind you supporting your weight. Place the foam roller under your calves (A). Slowly roll along the back of your legs up and down from your knees to your ankles (B).

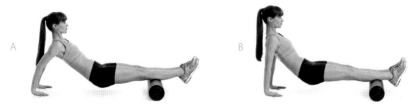

A

B

## → 2 HAMSTRINGS

Sit with your right leg on the roller; bend your left knee, cross your left ankle over your right ankle, and put your hands on the floor behind you (A). Roll up and down from your knee to just under your right butt cheek (B). Switch legs.

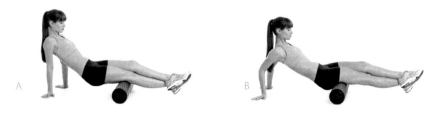

## → 3 QUADS

Lie facedown on the floor and place the roller under your hips (A). Lean on your left leg (B) and roll up and down from your hip to your knee. Switch legs.

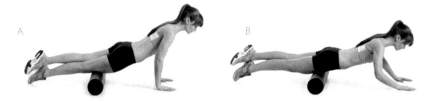

*A study in the* Journal of Strength and Conditioning Research *found that just 2 minutes of rolling is enough to improve recovery in quad muscles.*

## → 4 BACK

Sit on the floor with the foam roller on your lower back, resting your hands behind you for balance (A). Tighten your abs and slowly bend your knees to move the roller up your back, just below your shoulder blades (B).

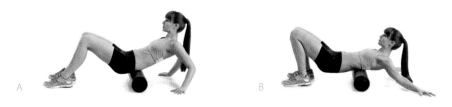

# ➜ 5 OUTER THIGHS

Lie on your side with the roller under your right hip (A). Bracing your abs and glutes for balance, slowly roll down from your hip to your knee (B). Switch to the other side and repeat.

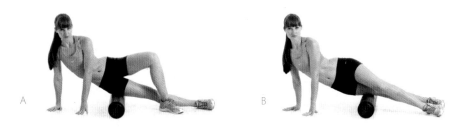

# ➜ 6 SHOULDERS AND SIDES

Lie on your back with the roller behind your shoulders. Lace your fingers loosely behind your head and lean your upper back into the roller (A). Brace your abs and glutes for stability, and slowly press into the roller on your left side, raising your right shoulder (B). Roll from your underarms to the bottom of your rib cage. Return to the center and switch sides.

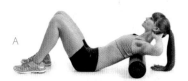
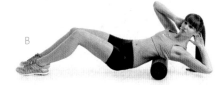

# ➜ 7 BUTT

Sitting on the roller, cross your right leg over your left knee and lean toward the right hip, putting your weight on your hands for support (A). Slowly roll one butt cheek over the roller (B). Switch sides.

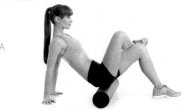
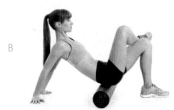

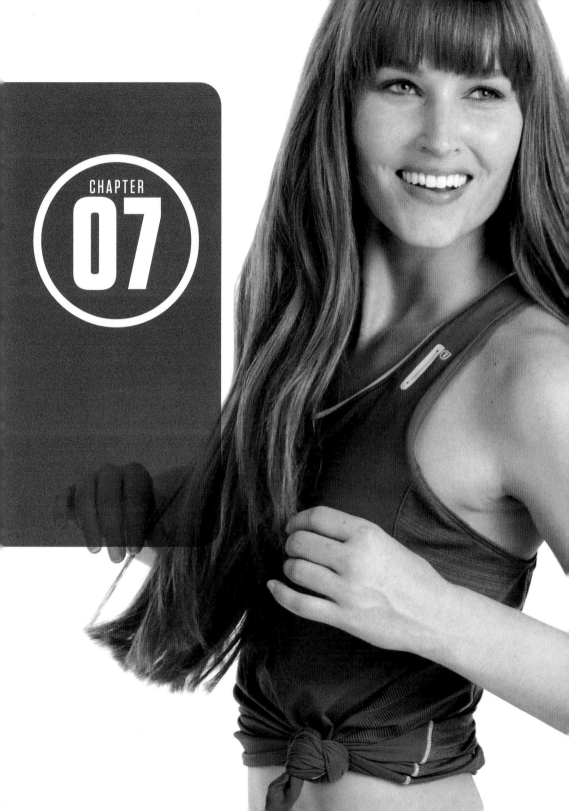

CHAPTER
**07**

# Crush More Calories

*Revamp your cardio routine for better results in less time*

**H**ere in America, you'll see rows of women sweating it out on treadmills (or ellipticals, stair steppers, or stationary bikes). Stop in again months later, and many of those same women won't look that much slimmer, despite the countless hours they've spent in those crowded cardio rooms.

While the logic behind "the more miles I log, the more weight I'll lose" may seem sound, there's a sneaky loophole. On the one hand, running is an incredibly effective form of exercise for burning calories. (You burn about 8.5 calories a minute when moving at a comfortable pace.) Problem is, when your body gets used to a routine, it becomes more efficient, so it uses less energy. Translation: You burn fewer calories and your gains in speed and endurance level off.

So while you may initially drop some pounds, your progress will flatline as soon as your body adjusts to a particular exercise regimen, which can cause many people to burn out and give up.

### SIMPLE ▶ SWAP

If you truly enjoy your long runs, rides, or swims, by all means, keep it up. If you're doing them to slim down, though, it's time to make a change: Replace one or two weekly long runs with any strength-training workout in Chapters 4 through 6, and one of the cardio workouts in this chapter. Then watch your results accelerate. You'll feel better and stronger—and look slimmer.

This chapter focuses on how to maximize aerobic exercise—yes, the "cardio" you know so well—by integrating fast, supercharged strategies that minimize your training time. Sorry to my distance runners, but you won't find slow-and-steady miles here. When it comes to fat loss, long-distance running is not your most efficient tool. I'm not saying you should abandon your marathon efforts—I'm only saying you don't *need* tons of mileage to lose weight and improve fitness. Instead, amp up your typical cardio routine and you'll see better results in record time.

# The Ultimate Weight-Loss Workout Zone

▶ For almost 2 decades, we've been hearing the seductive call of the "fat-burning zone," in which you burn a greater percentage of fat calories. And we've been told you get there by doing moderate—not hard—exercise.

Turns out, it's not that simple. When you exercise at 60 to 70 percent of your maximum heart rate, in that so-called zone, you burn fewer calories per minute during and after your workout. To crank your metabolism, you need to push your body harder—a lot harder.

Picture your physical activity level on a spectrum. On one end is the effortless kind, like sitting at your desk or walking to a meeting. When you're not exerting yourself, your body actually burns a higher percentage of calories from fat than it does when you're active. That's partly why the fat-burning zone was so appealing—it sounds awesome. But, of course, that doesn't mean sitting at your desk or wandering the halls at work will shrink your hips faster than doing jumping jacks or running a sprint.

Toward the other end of the activity spectrum is a super-intense workout that sends your heart rate way beyond the classic fat-burning zone. At this point, your body needs quick energy, so it starts burning less flab and turns instead to carbohydrates, which enter the bloodstream faster than fat does. The upside: The harder you work, the more calories you burn. At your max effort, experts estimate that you could be burning 20 to 30 calories a minute. And it's the total number of calories you burn that actually blasts body fat.

Besides burning more calories per minute, high-intensity exercise unleashes a flood of hormones, including epinephrine, which helps your body burn calories even when you're not working out. Case in point: People who cycled at a high intensity for 20 minutes torched more calories for hours after their workouts than they did after cycling at a low intensity for 30 to 60 minutes, according to a study reported in *Medicine & Science in Sports & Exercise*. You won't get those benefits from exercising in the classic fat-burning zone.

# Pick Up the Pace

➨ As it turns out, the new fat-burning zone isn't really a single zone at all. It's more like a cocktail of efforts that, when mixed together the right way, delivers a mega calorie crush to reveal a slimmer physique.

The one thing they all share: intensity. When you push on the gas pedal during your workouts, your body becomes less efficient and has to burn more calories to do the activity. Obviously, it's much harder to maintain that all-out effort for an extended period of time, which is why the best fat-fighting strategy is one that involves short bursts of activity that require you to breathe so hard you can't utter a word, followed by easier moves that let you catch your breath.

## PERSONAL SCORECARD

Not only are the workouts in this chapter ideal for busy schedules, but they also work no matter how fit you are. Base the intensity on your rate of perceived exertion (RPE), or how hard you feel like you're working (at 1, you can chat; at 10, you're unable to speak). Because your RPE will change as your fitness level improves, you can follow the same routine and continue to see results.

These quick-but-killer efforts may be the closest thing you'll find to a magic calorie-burning bullet. Not only do you spend less time working out (which is kinder to your body), you also continue to incinerate calories at an increased rate even during the walking or jogging recovery periods. This kind of training also builds muscle, prevents plateaus, and increases endurance. That's just the physical payoff: It also busts boredom, boosts confidence, and improves mental toughness, giving you the strength to keep going when your body wants to stop.

As valuable as high-intensity workouts are, a little goes a long way—and you don't want to OD on them. Adding extra speed more than once a week can increase your risk for injuries. Slip just one of these pace-pushing workout strategies into your weekly routine. And don't just stick with the one that feels easiest—it's best to mix and match various methods to keep your body guessing.

## TEMPOS

Think of tempos—maintaining a comfortably hard pace for a sustained period of time—as the little black dress of fitness. They're classic and they benefit everyone. They teach your body to use oxygen more efficiently by increasing your lactate threshold, or the point at which your body fatigues at a given pace. This means you can go longer and harder—and burn more calories—before feeling like you need to call it a day. The trick is to work just outside your comfort zone (or your "happy pace"). On a scale of 1 to 10 (1 being effortless, 10 being killer), you should feel like you're at a 7 or 8. At this speed, you're breathing heavily, but not so hard that you're gasping or have to stop.

**DO IT** After a warmup, increase your pace and hold it for 15 to 20 minutes, then finish with a 10-minute cooldown. If sustaining a tougher-than-normal effort for that long is painfully punishing, scale back: Hold the tempo pace for 5 minutes, then recover at an easy pace for 2 minutes. Repeat three times, then cool down.

*Quick tip: While running is a natural fit, you can apply these tactics to any cardio activity—elliptical workouts, cycling, even walking—so there's no excuse to skip a session.*

## INTERVALS

When you rotate high-intensity exercise (a 9 on that 1-to-10 scale) with recovery periods, you send your heart rate soaring and torch tons of calories. It's a fantastic strategy when you're pressed for time. In fact, a study published in the *Journal of Physiology* showed that short bursts of very intense exercise can produce the same results as traditional exercise. Translation: You're getting the benefits of a 60-minute workout in 30 minutes.

**DO IT** After a 10-minute warmup, speed up to an all-out effort for 30 seconds, then slow down to recover for 1 to 2 minutes. Beginners should work on repeating that pattern four to eight times, then cool down. As your fitness level increases, shorten your rest break to 1 minute and work up to doing 12 intervals total. (Find other intervals that are scientifically proven to shed flab fast on page 202.)

*Quick tip: Before you get into intervals, it's a good idea to get your body adjusted to the uptick in demand. Try this routine to get started: Find a soft surface (a track, a grass field, or a packed-sand beach) and put two markers about 30 to 40 yards apart. Start at one end and begin jogging, increasing your speed until you're crossing the other marker at an 8 or 9 effort level. Gently slow down and walk back to the start. Repeat for a total of 6 reps, adding reps each workout until you've done 10 to 12.*

## HILLS

Hill workouts increase your speed and power, improve your stamina, prevent overuse injuries (by engaging different muscles), and give you a gorgeous set of gams. Icing on the cake: For each degree of incline, experts say you can count on at least a 10 percent increase in calories burned. So running up a 5 percent grade (a gentle hill) will burn 50 percent more calories than running on a totally flat surface for the same amount of time.

But don't jump straight to a 5 percent incline on the treadmill—you'll hate it and never want to do it again. Start with a 2 to 3 percent incline (if you're outdoors, look for a gradual hill or incline—one that challenges you, but doesn't force you to stop or walk). It should feel challenging but manageable.

# TALK ABOUT INTENSITY!

Running experts have long referenced the "talk test" (how many words a person can spit out while hoofing it) as a way for people to gauge their efforts. Turns out, researchers have found it works for any aerobic exercise. (Okay, yes, it may be difficult while swimming.) This means, even if you're not following a workout with a set breakdown of RPEs (rates of perceived exertion), you can still make sure you're in the right training zone during every sweat session. Here's how to use the test—reciting the Pledge of Allegiance—for three different workout intensities.

### LOW-INTENSITY WARMUP

You should be able to say the entire pledge—all 31 words—comfortably, breathing at the usual pauses.
"I PLEDGE ALLEGIANCE TO THE FLAG OF THE UNITED STATES OF AMER-ICA . . . AND TO THE REPUBLIC FOR WHICH IT STANDS . . ."

### MODERATE AEROBIC ACTIVITY

Set a pace that allows you to easily recite four to six words at a time. You shouldn't have to strain to get the words out.
"I PLEDGE ALLEGIANCE TO THE FLAG . . . OF THE UNITED STATES OF AMERICA . . . AND TO THE REPUBLIC . . . FOR WHICH IT STANDS . . ."

### HIGH-INTENSITY INTERVALS

Sprint so you can say only a word or two between breaths. Recover until you can say the whole pledge comfortably.
"I PLEDGE . . . ALLEGIANCE . . . TO . . . THE FLAG . . . OF . . . THE UNITED . . . STATES . . . OF AMERICA . . ."

**DO IT** After warming up, ascend a hill at an even pace, then come back down to the base. Catch your breath (should be about 45 to 60 seconds) then repeat, working up to a total of 6 to 8 reps before cooling down. On a treadmill, you can either follow a programmed hill workout (choose level two or three) or create your own: Once you're warmed up, alternate running for 1 minute at a 2 to 3 percent grade with 1-minute recovery jogs at no incline. Work up to repeating this eight times, then finish with a 10-minute cooldown.

*Quick tip: Most people take an attack-and-conquer approach to hills, but hammering as hard as possible can cause you to burn out quickly. Instead, climb up at the same perceived effort (rather than pace) as your flat-terrain running. As you descend the hill, keep an even effort by speeding up.*

## PACES

If your to-do (or even wish) list includes a race, incorporating pace runs will help you get a feel for how fast you can go and still complete a certain distance in a given amount of time. If your goal is to finish a 5-K in 25 minutes, then you need to practice running at that pace to make sure it's doable on race day. Bonus benefit: These race-rehearsal sessions will burn more calories than a steady slog.

**DO IT** Pace workouts are based on the finish line you have in mind. For something like a 5-K, do 400-meter repeats: After a 10-minute warmup, run 400 meters (a quarter-mile, or one lap of a track) at your goal pace. Then jog or walk for 45 seconds. Build up to comfortably completing 10 repeats before race day.

*Repeats* is essentially a runner's term for intervals. You'll often see it used to describe speed workouts that refer to a specific distance, rather than a designated length of time.

# MIND MATTERS

**The urge to scream** "Uncle!" during a butt-kicking workout may have more to do with your overprotective brain than your cramping muscles. The traditional school of thought is that fatigue strikes when you're low on fuel, dehydrated, or overheated. But Timothy Noakes, MD, a professor of exercise and sports science at the University of Cape Town in South Africa, says that's not necessarily the case. "Before you even start working out, your brain is figuring out how to pace your body so that you stop exercising long before you have an issue," he says. Translation: You always have more in the tank than your brain leads you to believe.

While the world's most hard-driving athletes know how to ignore that fake-out and get more from their bodies, most of us can't help but fixate on our achy legs and burning lungs. But if that's all you think about, your brain can produce a stress response that increases the ache.

Our experience of pain is very much connected to our perception of it. If you decide the pain is unbearable, your tolerance for it will be lower than if you think you can handle it. So give yourself a mental pep talk before you hop on the treadmill. Remind yourself of how strong and capable you are.

But what if that bring-it-on attitude turns meek when the hurt sets in? Try one of these research-backed tricks: Mentally repeat the word *smooth* with each pedal stroke on a bike or continuously count up to eight during a run (known as rhythmic cognitive behavior), sing a favorite song or go over your grocery list (distraction or dissociation), or remind yourself that this sprint or strength-training interval will be over in just 30 more seconds (establishing an end).

# 8 Fat-Blasting Cardio Workouts

▶ Based on the techniques you just read about, these programs may look simple—but they'll kick your metabolism into hyperdrive in less than 30 minutes.

## 1. The Mile Challenge

Want to set a new personal record at your next race? Or just want a workout that kicks your ass and tests (better yet, improves) your max speed? Then try this workout from Bill Hartman, PT, CSCS, co-owner of Indianapolis Fitness and Sports Training.

1. Break down the total distance into smaller increments and calculate the speed required at each in order to complete the entire distance at your desired pace. So if you want to run a 6-minute mile, you have to be able to run . . .
   - a half-mile in 3 minutes
   - a quarter-mile in 90 seconds
   - 200 meters in 45 seconds
   - 100 meters in 22.5 seconds
2. Run a repeat at the longest distance you can make the time. (Can't make the 100-meter time? Readjust your per-mile pace.)
3. Rest three times as long as the length of the interval (so for 200 meters, that's 2 minutes and 15 seconds).
4. Continue the repeats until you can no longer maintain 90 percent of the speed. (Figure it out by dividing the time by 0.9. So 200-meter repeats are continued until you can no longer make it in 50 seconds.)

## 2. Cardio Climber

Try this "ladder" interval drill, climbing up (run gradually longer intervals) or down (run gradually shorter intervals): Run 1 minute hard, 2 minutes easy, 2 minutes hard, 3 minutes easy, 3 minutes hard, 4 minutes easy, and then work back down.

## 3. Flip On Your Fat Burners

The problem with interval workouts: Some are so complicated you can't remember them! This one couldn't get any easier—to remember, that is. Researchers found that people who followed a program similar to this one three times a week for 2 weeks saw the same benefits as those who completed 10 hours of moderate exercise during the 2 weeks. In layman's terms: You'll improve your body's efficiency in one-fifth of the time.

After a short warmup, complete the following workout, repeating the pattern 10 times. Finish with a 3- to 5-minute cooldown.

### *ON* Sprint!

For 1 minute, run at a pace that leaves you winded, but not breathless. (Think 8 out of 10, with 10 being your top speed.)

### *OFF* Recover!

For 1 minute, jog or walk. (You should be able to speak comfortably by the end.)

## 4. 20-Minute Tempos

**0-5 minutes:** *Warmup* (easy effort; you can sing at this pace)

**5-7 minutes:** *Moderate effort* (you can carry on a conversation)

**7-10 minutes:** *Hard effort* (you can speak only a few words at a time)

**10-12 minutes:** *Moderate effort*

**12-14 minutes:** *Recovery* (easy effort)

**14-16 minutes:** *Very hard effort* (you're huffing and puffing too much to talk)

**16-20 minutes:** *Cooldown* (easy effort)

# 5. Speed Booster

Many speed workouts come with two training speeds—superfast or barely moving. This plan adds a third, moderate speed into each 1-minute interval segment. This tweak actually helps exercisers maintain a higher heart rate for longer, which builds endurance and speed faster, according to researchers. In fact, a study published in the *Journal of Applied Physiology* reported that exercisers who followed this routine for 20 to 30 minutes were able to drop a minute off their 5-K times. (But you can gain similar benefits from just 12 minutes.) Start with a short warmup, follow this 30-20-10 plan, then finish with a short cooldown.

**0:00–0:30** Jog at a slow pace

**0:31–0:50** Run at a moderate pace

**0:51–1:00** Sprint

**1:01–5:00** Repeat the 30-20-10 interval (five times total)

**5:01–6:59** Walk

**7:00–7:30** Jog at a slow pace

**7:31–7:50** Run at a moderate pace

**7:51–8:00** Sprint

**8:01–12:00** Repeat the 30-20-10 interval (five times total)

# 6. Buildup Basics

Use this template for a tempo plan that revs up your metabolism anytime, anywhere.

**2 Minutes:** *Easy–Moderate* (4 out of 10 intensity level)

**2 Minutes:** *Moderate* (5 out of 10 intensity)

**1 Minute:** *Hard* (8 out of 10 intensity)

# X 3

**+ 5 Minutes:** *Easy* (3 out of 10 intensity)

# 7. Calorie-Shredding Shuttle

This deceptively simple cardio drill will raise your heart rate and incinerate calories. Find 30 feet of open space and place three markers in a line, each 15 feet away from the other. Straddling the middle marker, sprint to your right and touch the line with your right hand. Immediately turn and sprint back to your left for 30 feet and touch with your left hand; turn once more and sprint back to your starting point. That's 1 rep (it should take 5 to 7 seconds). Rest for 25 seconds, and on your next rep, move to your left first. Continue this pattern until you complete 10 reps.

 **SLIM-DOWN SECRET**

Cramming in your cardio? Stretch after—not before—to go farther and faster, report Florida State University researchers. Subjects who didn't loosen up prior to a 30-minute treadmill run logged an extra 220 yards compared with those who stretched for more than 15 minutes beforehand. Normally, muscle fibers are like tight rubber bands, springing your legs off the ground faster so your feet move quicker. Stretching lengthens these fibers, making them less elastic and slower to react. Instead, study authors recommend warming up with a 5- to 10-minute jog or brisk walk.

# 8. Run Your Butt Off!

Even though I'm stressing short-and-sweet cardio workouts and that you don't *need* a full-fledged cardio plan, I know some of you don't want to ditch your running routine. I get it. That's why I've included this simple but efficient 8-week weight-loss program created by Andrew Kastor, head coach at Mammoth Track Club in Mammoth Lakes, California (and, yes, husband of three-time Olympian Deena Kastor). Good news: You don't need to log more than one long run a week (meaning 30 minutes or more). This sustained effort will improve your endurance by increasing your heart's capacity and strengthening ligaments and tendons, so you feel stronger during your short runs.

## BEGINNER

**MONDAY** 20- to 30-minute cross training + strength

Strength workouts should be mostly total body, or focused on core and lower body. (Use any of the workouts in this book.)

**TUESDAY** Interval workout

Run hard for 15 to 30 seconds, jog or walk for 60 seconds. Repeat 6 times, building up to 10 over 8 weeks.

**WEDNESDAY** Off

**THURSDAY** Hills (optional)

On a gentle hill (or up to 5 percent on treadmill), run hard for 10 seconds, then walk down or recover for up to 60. Repeat 4 to 8 times.

**FRIDAY** 20- to 30-minute cross training + strength

**SATURDAY** 4-minute easy run/1-minute walk for 15 minutes

Each week, add 5 minutes to your Saturday run/walk. At Week 4, go back to this starting point and build up by 5-minute increments again.

**SUNDAY** Off

## EXPERIENCED

**MONDAY** Strength + 20- to 30-minute run

**TUESDAY** Interval workout

Follow the same workout as the beginner program; but build up to 12 total.

**WEDNESDAY** Off

**THURSDAY** Hills

Complete the same hill workout above, but repeat 6 to 10 times.

**FRIDAY** Strength + (optional) 20- to 30-minute run

**SATURDAY** 30- to 60-minute run, depending on your typical mileage

Each week, add 5 minutes to your Saturday run (if you're starting at 60 minutes, add 2 minutes). At Week 4, go back to Saturday's starting point and build up again.

**SUNDAY** Off

# Get into Top Form

➦ Just like with strength training, proper form during aerobic exercise is crucial. This cheat sheet will help you do it better—whether you're running, biking, swimming, or on the elliptical or stair stepper.

## Stride Right

Running with good form will keep your body happy and out of the doctor's office. Sharpen your step with these simple form pointers.

- *Fast feet.* Take quick, short steps instead of longer strides, which can hurt your lower back and tire you out. Your feet should land under your center of gravity, not out in front of you.
- *Soft steps.* Land lightly between your heel and midfoot, and let your foot roll smoothly forward. Push off with your toes.
- *Head up.* Look ahead and scan the horizon to prevent slouching (unless you're running on a trail or other bumpy surface).
- *Straight swing.* Relax your arms and bend them about 90 degrees, letting them swing front to back (not across your midline) between waist and lower-chest level. Keep your hands loose—think about lightly holding a piece of paper between your thumb and pointer finger.
- *Lean in.* Lean forward from your hips to maintain momentum without sacrificing your posture. (To get the approximate feel, stand still on both feet, then shift your weight toward the balls of your feet without lifting your heels.)
- *Proud chest.* Keep your chest lifted, shoulders stretching down your back. Imagine there is a string attached to your sternum pulling you upward as you run.

# GET BACK ON THE ROAD

Like I've said, running is not a requirement for fat loss; however, it is an incredibly accessible tool (no equipment required but you and your sneakers!). But if you're a beginning runner (or it's been 6 months or longer since you ran anything over a mile), ramping up your mileage or speed too quickly can book you an express ticket back to the sidelines.

The best thing you can do is start out slowly—really slowly. Easing into it helps your muscles get used to the impact of running and helps your mind get used to the effort. Use this run/walk program three times a week (on nonconsecutive days). Begin and end each session with a 5-minute warmup walk. Repeat a week if you don't feel ready to move up. The sign you're ready to start tacking on more mileage (and eventually, speed): You can run consistently for at least 30 minutes.

**WEEK 1:**
Run 2 minutes, walk 3 minutes;
REPEAT 6 TIMES

**WEEK 2:**
Run 3 minutes, walk 3 minutes;
REPEAT 5 TIMES

**WEEK 3:**
Run 5 minutes, walk 2 minutes;
REPEAT 4 TIMES

**WEEK 4:**
Run 7 minutes, walk 3 minutes;
REPEAT 4 TIMES

**WEEK 5:**
Run 8 minutes, walk 2 minutes;
REPEAT 3 TIMES

**WEEK 6:**
Run 9 minutes, walk 1 minute;
REPEAT 3 TIMES

**WEEK 7:**
Run 30 minutes

# Spin Doctors

Whether you're in spin class or out on the road, there's a better way to ride your two-wheeler. Put these tips to use to get fitter and stave off injury.

- *Pedal smoothly.* Your goal: Cycle in fluid circles rather than jamming down on the pedals. To do this, push down on the pedal with the ball of your foot; next, pull your foot through the bottom of the stroke, then pull up and back around. Aim for about 90 rpm (to calculate rpm, count how many times your right knee comes up in 60 seconds).
- *Eyes on the prize.* Resist the urge to put your head down when you're going hard or getting tired. It can slow your oxygen intake, tiring you out faster. (Not to mention that on the road, it spells danger.)
- *Core performance.* While your legs are busy pumping, keep your upper body still—don't rock side to side, especially while climbing. Maintain a flat back and keep your elbows bent and relaxed (it helps absorb shock when you hit a bump outside). Hold your arms in line with your body, not out to the side. Keeping your upper body relaxed will reduce strain on your lower back.
- *Take a seat.* Your weight should feel evenly distributed, with 60 percent on the saddle (seat) and 40 percent on the handlebar. The saddle height should be positioned so there's a slight bend in your knee when your foot is at the bottom of a stroke. Most of all, you should be comfortable. Your best bet? Get a professional bike fit at a shop.
- *Get up.* Sitting is the most efficient way to ride—you can use up to 10 percent more energy when you're out of the saddle. But sometimes, like on a monster hill, you need extra power. When you stand, all of your body weight pushes down on the pedals, giving each stroke more oomph. If you stand, shift into a harder gear so your legs don't circle too quickly, rise up, and keep your butt over the seat.

# BIKE YOUR WAY TO A BETTER BODY

Cycling is a multitasking cardio workout that fries fat and demolishes stress without pounding you into the ground. Here's how it can make you a lean, fat-burning machine.

### It Torches Calories.

Even pedaling at an easy pace, a 130-pound woman will torch 473 calories in an hour. Upping the speed to 14 to 16 mph burns close to 591 calories.

### It Sculpts Killer Legs.

Your quads, glutes, and calves are keeping you moving. To better engage these muscles, focus on your pedal stroke. Try to make a perfect circle: Push forward and then down with your quads; pull back with your hamstrings, as if you're wiping mud off the bottom of your shoe; and then use your calves and hip flexors to pull up and back.

### It Saves Your Joints.

Riding a bike puts a lot less stress on the knees, ankles, and spine than walking or running. This means you can develop muscle power and cardio endurance without feeling the same impact.

### It Tones All Over.

It's not just your legs that benefit: Pedaling while standing engages your core and triceps as you stabilize your body over the bike. Spend roughly half the time pedaling out of the saddle, focusing on keeping your core tight.

### It Protects Your Ticker.

Heart disease is the number-one killer of women in this country, and two top risk factors are high blood pressure and high LDL cholesterol. In one study, researchers had 32 women ride at a moderate to high intensity three times a week for at least half an hour. After a year, they'd lowered their blood pressure and LDL, as well as significantly increased their aerobic fitness.

# Step Right Up

There's a reason the stair stepper is a cardio machine mainstay in most gyms: It's not only a big-time calorie scorcher; it also sculpts your hips, legs, and butt without taking a toll on your body (the way some other machines can).

There's just one problem. Most women make fundamental mistakes that cost them the hot-body results they're after. To make the most of your time on the stepper, keep these tips in mind.

- **Straighten up.** Your body should form a straight line; keep it upright with your hips centered over your legs. (Many women hunch forward or stick their butts out.)
- **Skip the support.** Either place your hands gently on the machine, elbows bent at 90 degrees, or by your sides, moving back and forth as if you're running.
- **Step solid.** Press your entire heel down on the step. This forces your glutes and hamstrings to work, instead of just the calf muscles. But avoid pushing the step all the way down or letting it come all the way up. This can make your pelvis sway up and down, which can lead to soreness and injury.
- **Zone in.** Form slips when your mind drifts. Stay focused on squeezing your glutes every time your heel presses into the step.

# Dive In

Swimming is one of the best workouts for torching fat and trimming inches. The body-shaping benefits of swimming are the result of a perfect storm of calorie burn and muscle recruitment. Because water is nearly 800 times denser than air, each kick, push, and pull is like a mini resistance workout for your entire body—especially your core, hips, arms, shoulders, and glutes. So not only are you blasting calories (an easy swim burns around 500 calories an hour, while a vigorous effort can torch almost 700), but you also build lean muscle and boost your metabolism.

Synchronize your basic freestyle stroke with these tips.

- **Keep your head down.** Align your head and neck with your spine, and keep your shoulders relaxed. Look at the black line on the bottom of the pool with your head in a neutral position. This will prevent your hips from sinking and keep your body level in the water.
- **Roll over.** As you rotate your body to the side to breathe, rotate your head (don't lift it out of the water) and take a breath through your mouth. Exhale gently and gradually under the water until your next breath.
- **Do arm circles.** Pull through the water, keeping your fingers pointed toward the bottom of the pool. Your hand should trace an imaginary line on the pool's bottom. Finish each stroke by extending your arm fully behind you until your hand is close to your thigh.
- **Open your hands.** Avoid cupping your hands. When they're relaxed, with your fingers slightly open, they'll propel you forward more easily.
- **Keep your elbows up.** Your elbows should always be higher than your wrist.
- **Use your hips.** The kick starts in the hips and core. Imagine you're trying to kick off a pair of flip-flops in the water.
- **Kick it with fast feet.** Keep your feet close together and in line with the rest of your body. They should be pointed naturally, fluttering at about six kicks per stroke.

# DIFFERENT STROKES

**Freestyle is a fan favorite** because it's easy to learn and burns major calories. But it pays to mix things up. Using various strokes balances your muscles and helps beat boredom. Two to try are backstroke (it improves your posture by working your back and shoulder muscles) and breaststroke (it uses the hip and inner-thigh muscles, which are often missed in other workouts). Use these quick tips to get more from each stroke.

## Backstroke

### Eyes up.
Look straight up at the sky or ceiling—not at your toes, which causes your hips to sink—so your head is in line with your spine.

### Make a Y.
Reach back with each arm at a 45-degree angle to your body; it places less stress on your shoulders and makes your stroke stronger.

## Breaststroke

### Sweep through.
Reach your arms overhead, palms together. Rotating your palms outward, pull down until your hands are nearly level with your chin. Bring your hands inward by your chest, then reach again.

### Whip it.
Bend your knees and bring your heels toward your butt. Turn your toes outward and kick your legs back and together (like a frog) as you extend your arms forward.

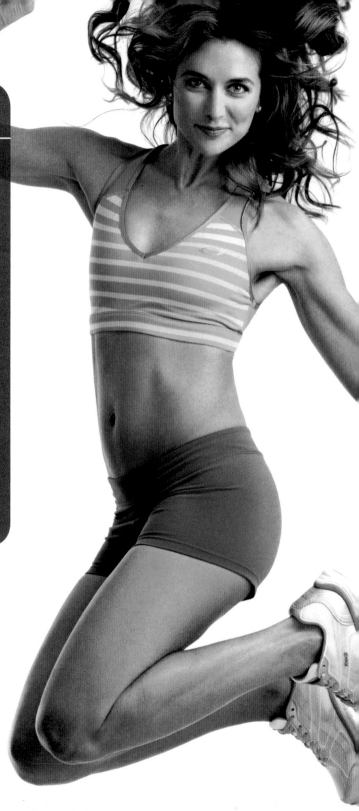

# Look Hot in a Hurry

*Tackle any weight-loss deadline—without going nuts*

Nothing seems to ignite healthier eating or super-dedicated work-outs more than deadlines—especially when they involve break-ing out a bikini or looking better than ever at a reunion.

Getting into great shape can be daunting enough; doing it with ambitious weight-loss goals or tight time frames raises the bar even higher—and the extra pressure is not always productive. Most women trade in *moderate* and *consistent* for *agonizing* and *excessive*. They jump off the couch and into the gym for hours of cardio and drastically cut back calories.

It hurts. It sucks. It zaps most of their time and almost all of their energy. But if it *feels* like they're closing in on their goals, it somehow seems worth it.

More often than not, though, the plan backfires and these women fall short of their goals. Even if—for the sake of argument—they succeed, there's a high probability their approach is setting them up for future failure.

For starters, in-a-rush dieting causes many women to overlook impor-tant cues, like fatigue and pain. Ignoring muscle soreness or tightness is like continuing to drive your car when the check-engine light flashes on the dashboard: It just sets you up for bigger problems and potentially serious injuries. What's more, when you don't exercise regularly, bursts of intense activity require your heart and lungs to work much harder than they are used to.

The out-the-door sprint almost always leads to slacking off and moti-vational burnout, too. As soon as the big event is over, you take a vaca-tion from your extreme regimen. After all, you "deserve" it for all your hard work. Two missed workouts snowball into 2 months of missed workouts, and suddenly you can't button your jeans or do a pushup to save your life. In fact, research shows that body fat, weight, and waist size can rise—and fitness levels can dip—after just a 5-week hiatus.

# Score the Body You Want in Record Time

▶ While weight loss seems like a relatively straightforward equation—calories in have to be less than calories out—each deadline has its own subtle but unique approach for delivering results. For example, cardio at a steady, moderate pace can help a woman who is 20 pounds overweight kick off her fitness program and see early results. But try that approach when you're single digits away from your goal and your results will likely flatline. Similarly, while someone with 2 weeks until her vacation can pick up the intensity or frequency at the gym, doing so 6 weeks out can lead to early burnout or injury. The most effective time-crunched strategy should be tailored to your situation (the reason you fell off the wagon to begin with, like an injury or a hectic work schedule); the amount of time you have till your big event; the number of pounds you need to lose; and what kind of shape you're currently in. How quickly you can hit your desired target depends on a number of individual factors, but the common denominator is avoiding the fitness and diet mistakes that can wind up slowing you down—or even sidelining you. Throughout this chapter, you'll find solutions for getting where you want to go—as quickly as possible. Use the tips that match your time frame and goals to help you work out more effectively and pace yourself for fast, but not fleeting, results.

## Your Trim-Down Timeline

Before starting any successful weight-loss program, you need an accurate and realistic frame of reference for how long it will take to *burn body fat*. Notice that I didn't say *lose weight*. Though often used interchangeably, these two things are not mutually exclusive. (You can, in fact, lose weight at a much faster pace—by shedding water weight and sometimes even precious fat-fighting lean muscle.) Your trim-down timeline depends on a variety of factors, including your age, gender, activity level, calories consumed, and your current weight, which means your pace is going to be individualized. Keep in mind that while people with more weight to lose can see larger losses almost immediately, seeing double-digit drops like TV weight-loss contestants isn't realistic. (And it's a good sign you're losing weight, not body fat.) Of course, we all want the quickest fix, but that immediate gratification pales in comparison to actually maintaining the weight loss for years after. A typical barometer for fat loss is losing up to 2 pounds a week.

## SLIM-DOWN SECRET

It can be tempting to weigh in every day, but you shouldn't. For starters, the scale can't take into account that you dropped body fat but added metabolism-boosting lean muscle mass. It's also easily swayed by daily (if not hourly) fluctuations in your water and food intake. In short, frequent weigh-ins don't always paint an accurate picture of how you're doing. If you can't stay off the scale, use it once a week. Researchers found that overweight people who weigh themselves about once a week are six times more likely to lose weight. It helps to do it on the same day and generally the same time every week. I recommend Monday morning: Knowing you're going to be measuring your progress at the start of the week can help many women make better decisions (or at least be more conscious about the ones they're making) throughout the weekend.

*"A goal is a dream with a deadline."*

—NAPOLEON HILL

# The Fastest Way to Lose . . .

## 20+ Pounds

Your goal weight may seem far off, but don't sweat it. The more you weigh, the more calories you burn during easier workouts like brisk walking. No need for killer workouts just yet: Small, consistent efforts will help you shed pounds early on—and seeing those quick results will motivate you to stay on track.

### STRENGTH PRESCRIPTION: STAY OFF THE SIDELINE

Your biggest challenge is keeping injuries at bay. Excess weight makes exercise naturally harder on your joints. Start with basic bodyweight exercises 2 days a week; they put less strain on your body and help you learn proper form. "The Greatest Bodyweight Workout Ever" on page 152 is built to adjust with you; once you master the fundamental moves, your joints and muscles will be prepped to tackle more-difficult exercises and increase to three sessions per week.

### CARDIO PRESCRIPTION: NICE AND EASY

In most cases slow and steady isn't the best approach, but it's the key to developing endurance, a crucial building block at this weight-loss stage. Sustained, moderate-intensity cardio slowly introduces your joints to impact, reducing your risk of getting injured. What's more, it helps teach

## # BY THE NUMBERS

**22**
Percentage of weight loss that comes from losing muscle when dieters don't lift weights, according to Pennsylvania State University researchers.

your body to utilize fat as fuel so that over time you begin to burn more of it. Two days a week, aim to complete 30 to 45 minutes of easy- to moderate-intensity cardio (you can walk, hike, bike, or swim—anything that keeps you going for at least 30 minutes). Mix up your routine to train different muscles and beat boredom. And pay attention to your body: It's better to do too little than too much at this stage. If you're feeling fatigued, lower the duration of a workout or take a day off.

## 10 Pounds

Breaking this double-digit barrier can be frustrating. Your body adapts to exercise over time, which can cause your metabolism to fall into a lull. So if you were seeing steady results and then hit a point of slow or stalled progress, your body likely adapted to the stimulus. In short: Your body got fitter, and now your go-to routine won't cut it.

### STRENGTH PRESCRIPTION: PUT ON WEIGHT

Repeat after me: The secret to sailing into double digits is strength training three times a week—and not with 3-pound dumbbells. Adding resistance helps you torch more calories during and after your workout while replacing body fat with lean muscle mass. It's important to track your progress during workouts. When you hit a plateau, increase one of these four things: frequency (so go from three workouts a week to four); intensity (if you've been using 10-pound dumbbells, go up to 15);

*"It's never too late to be who you might have been."*

—GEORGE ELIOT

time (increase your workout duration by 5 minutes); or type (if you've been doing the same routine, or taking the same Pilates class, switch it up).

 **2-SECOND LIFE CHANGER**

*Sweat incentives.* Having a supportive training buddy or class instructor can increase your workout's effectiveness. According to researchers, receiving verbal praise during your workout can actually help you perform exercises even better next time. It seems to activate the same reward circuits in the brain as major incentives (like cash) and help solidify your muscle memory for that particular skill.

## CARDIO PRESCRIPTION: PICK UP THE TEMPO

Now that your body is ready, dial up your cardio with tempos—longer intervals done at a moderately difficult intensity (which I touched on in Chapter 7). The goal is sustained intensity—not overall duration (translation: burning more calories in less time). A good gauge you're in the right zone: You should be able to talk, but not easily.

# 5 Pounds

It's a pretty cruel joke if you ask me: The closer you get to your ideal weight, the tougher it is to reach it. Your body is always working to maintain its natural balance, so the more weight you lose, the harder your body works to hold on to it.

## STRENGTH PRESCRIPTION: TURN UP THE ENERGY

One way to shake your body out of its comfort zone is with plyometrics. These explosive moves are great muscle builders, get your heart rate up, and work multiple muscles at a time. That's what makes this megawatt routine the final piece of your weight-loss puzzle: It'll shed that last layer of fat to show off the sculpted, lean physique you've been building all along. Try the "1-Minute Burpee Challenge!" on page 144 or the workout in "Step Up Your Results" on page 174.

## CARDIO PRESCRIPTION: FAST AND FURIOUS

To beat plateaus and kick your fat-burning potential into overdrive, make your cardio as explosive as your strength training. As you may remember from Chapter 7, high-intensity interval training involves quick, sprintlike bursts combined with periods of rest or easy recovery to help maximize your calorie burn. In other words, go as close to all-out as you can. Twice a week, complete an interval using the cardio of your choice. (Find options in Chapter 7.) Feeling good? Boost your weekly calorie burn with an extra day of cardio—30 to 45 minutes at moderate intensity (or 65 to 80 percent of your maximum heart rate).

**SLIM-DOWN** SECRET

Research shows there's a surprising connection between elevating your mood and shedding stubborn pounds. One of the most important tips for successful weight loss is not to let past failed attempts keep you from trying again.

*"Do not wait for ideal circumstances nor for the best opportunities; they will never come."*

—JANET ERSKINE STUART

# RATE YOUR BURN

Kicking ass at boot camp or during your treadmill sprints does no good if it lands you on the couch for the rest of the day—or week. Paying attention to how you feel, particularly your soreness and energy level, turns out to be a pretty accurate gauge of how prepared your body is for your next workout, according to a study in the *Journal of Strength and Conditioning Research*. Use this scale to decide how hard you should push yourself next time:

| | | |
|---|---|---|
| *If your muscles ache and you feel completely wiped out:* | **Rate yourself a . . .** 1 or 2 (very poorly or not well recovered). | **Today you should . . .** Take a rest day or do a light active-recovery workout (go for a walk; do some yoga or foam rolling). |
| *If you're a little stiff and tired, but you feel generally strong:* | **Rate yourself a . . .** 5 or 6 (somewhat to moderately recovered). | **Today you should . . .** Go ahead with your regularly scheduled workout, but pay attention. If a specific move or speed causes discomfort, back off. |
| *If you feel fresh, energized, and ready to go:* | **Rate yourself a . . .** 9 or 10 (very well or completely recovered). | **Today you should . . .** Feel free to amp up your workout—push the pace 20 percent harder or go 20 percent longer during cardio. |

# Look Your Best in . . .

## 6 Weeks

Write out a manageable schedule you can stick to for at least 5 weeks. A study in *Health Psychology* reports that it takes new exercisers that long to make their sessions a habit. To prevent burnout, aim for consistent (4 to 5 days a week), moderate workouts. Too many days off in between workouts can decrease drive, especially when your deadline feels so far away. Cap each session at 30 minutes to make sure your muscles can recover. "Transform Your Body— In 24 Minutes!" in Chapter 4 is the perfect fit: 20-minute workouts that check off strength training and cardio, three times per week.

**2-SECOND LIFE CHANGER**

Invest in some form-fitting workout clothes. According to researchers at Springfield College in Massachusetts, most new exercisers typically go for baggy clothes. But the excess fabric hampers movement, which can make them feel even worse about themselves.

**FOOD FOR THOUGHT:** Think *replace* rather than *trim*. Cutting calories too drastically this far out can feel too taxing. Instead, make one replacement during each meal to get more nutrients like healthy fats, fiber, and protein into your diet. It's as simple as sprinkling your yogurt with flaxseed at breakfast, or adding a handful of fresh spinach to your pasta sauce at dinner.

## 4 Weeks

Same basic rules apply at 4 weeks, especially if you're a beginner or it's been a few months since you've last worked out. In fact, people in these categories will likely struggle the most with this time frame: managing their eagerness for lightning-fast results, while giving their body enough of a break-in period to adjust to the new routine before dialing up the intensity. Use the same "Transform Your Body—In 24 Minutes" workout from Chapter 4, but focus on two areas of your execution: load and tempo. You'll get the best results by choosing a weight that really challenges you to finish the set. At the same time, complete each rep as fast as possible with good form, only stopping briefly when your form falters.

**FOOD FOR THOUGHT:** Consider yourself a B student when it comes to your diet and follow the 80-20 rule. About 80 percent of the foods you eat should be lean protein, such as poultry, fish, and beans; fruits and vegetables; low-fat dairy; high-fiber grain products; and healthier fats such as olive oil. The other 20 percent can be foods that are not as healthy.

## 2 Weeks

This may be the one time that balls-to-the-wall motivation and dedication can work in your favor. In this short window, it's easier to stay dialed in and committed; plus, your body can tolerate a few extra sweat sessions—*if* you train smart. Supercharge your metabolism by choosing any three strength workouts in this book and add two high-intensity intervals per week (find options in Chapter 7). Whenever you dial up the intensity, it's important to keep an eye on the overall impact: To keep injuries at bay, choose at least one low-impact cardio choice (like swimming and cycling) each week.

**FOOD FOR THOUGHT:** Cut back on carbs. It's one of the most reliable strategies for short-term weight loss. Case in point: Dutch researchers found that eating one carb-free meal a day over a 2-week period can increase metabolic rate by 81 calories per day. The key is making the

## 2-SECOND LIFE CHANGER

When your big event has come and gone, don't lay off your routine completely. Even taking just 1 week off can cause you to slide. Give your body (and mind) a break by scaling back your weekly routine by 30 to 50 percent for the next week (or if you're really drained, two). So, if you were doing three strength workouts and 2 days of cardio, cut back to two strength workouts (and one cardio workout, if you're feeling up to it). Shorter sessions count, too: Try any of the "5-Minute Fat Blasters" in Chapter 5, starting on page 118.

meal about 70 percent protein, and, of course, zero carbs. (Watch for sneaky carb sources like milk, sausages, and barbecue sauce—just to name a few.)

## 1 Week

It may sound counterintuitive, but scaling back your workout frequency and intensity could help keep you on track. Keep your routine light and manageable—walk 10,000 steps each day and complete one or two light strength-training workouts each week. While doing tons of cardio will undoubtedly burn extra calories, it could also ramp up your appetite.

**FOOD FOR THOUGHT:** There's no sense in starving. Eventually, you'll end up breaking down and overeating. Follow the "7 Days to Slim" plan opposite to make smart and targeted changes.

# The 4 Stages of Exercise Burnout

➤ Like sleep, grief, and relationships, exercise—or more accurately, exercise burnout—has classic stages. You're always in one of the four stages, but moving between them doesn't happen overnight and people

# 7 DAYS TO SLIM

Implement one simple tweak every day (and keep it up till the big day) to feel lighter and firmer in just 1 week.

**SUNDAY Eliminate processed foods**
If you can't pronounce the ingredients, the food is off-limits. Or hit the produce aisle for foods with no label at all.

**MONDAY Lay off the sauce**
Not only are alcoholic drinks dehydrating and high in calories, they also make resisting nibbles difficult. (No shocker here: Studies prove women consume more calories after drinking.)

**TUESDAY Get a fiber fix**
It may be tempting to nix all carbs, but don't forgo fiber, a proven source of long-lasting satiety. Sprinkle flaxseed onto yogurt or add a few teaspoons of sliced almonds to your salad.

**WEDNESDAY Burn, baby, burn**
Eating steadily throughout the day can prevent hunger—which makes you want to ravage anything in sight.

Aim for three small meals (300 to 350 calories each) and two snacks (100 to 150 calories each).

**THURSDAY Banish bloat**
Broccoli, onions, and peppers cause gassiness and bloating. Stick to water-based produce like cucumbers, spinach, and asparagus. Potassium-rich fruits like bananas and oranges also purge retained water.

**FRIDAY Flush it out**
Cells retain water when they don't have enough of it. Down 2 to 3 liters each day. Sip slowly and the water will hit your bloodstream rather than filter out through your liver, so you won't have to pee every 5 seconds.

**THE BIG DAY! Befriend protein**
A healthy, protein-rich breakfast will fill you up and head off unnecessary snacking. Try one of the lightning-fast egg recipes on page 267.

typically don't pass through them at the same rate. Clue into the classic symptoms—and tips for how to stay on track—so you can sidestep a workout slump.

## Stage 1 The Honeymoon

You're determined to look hot at your best friend's wedding, so you ramp up your workouts to 6 or 7 days a week—and you never miss a single session.

**STAY ON TRACK:** Take a less-is-more approach. Burnout often happens

# LOOK BETTER TOMORROW!

**Last-minute weekend plans?** Don't expect miracles, but here's what celebrity trainer Valerie Waters advises her clients to do in a pinch.

***Get moving.*** Torch calories and spike your metabolism with a 20-minute, fast-paced strength circuit using light resistance (or just your body weight).

***Cut it out.*** Say no to sugar, alcohol, sodium, and refined carbs (such as white bread and pasta), and limit fiber intake to about 25 grams a day. All of this stuff causes your body to retain water, making you look (and feel) bloated.

***Dine in.*** This dinner combination revs up your metabolism and helps eliminate extra water weight: 4 ounces of low-fat fish (such as halibut, cod, or tilapia) drizzled with a flavorful low-fat spinach sauce (blend two large handfuls of spinach, 2 teaspoons olive oil, and lemon juice to taste in a blender until smooth). Serve with a side of roasted, nonstarchy vegetables, such as green beans.

when you expect too much too soon, so balance your excitement with the big picture. Even with the smartest, most effective workout program, you still can't force your body to become stronger or slimmer any faster than it physiologically can. Don't exceed your ability to recover mentally or physically: Start with the lowest reps, sets, and weights. Gradually increase exercise volume and intensity to avoid injury; and always pencil in at least one full day off. (Recovery days are essential—you'll hear more about that in the following chapter.)

## # BY THE NUMBERS

## 10

Number of additional reps people could complete while listening to their favorite music, according to a study from the College of Charleston in South Carolina.

## Stage 2 Disenchantment

Your excitement fades when you don't see results right away. You stop looking forward to gym time and start slacking during—or flat-out skipping—workouts.

**STAY ON TRACK:** Find support. According to Penn State researchers, simply having a supportive friend, family member, or significant other makes you more likely to stick with your fitness regimen. Participants who started a new workout plan with a partner cheering

 **2-SECOND LIFE CHANGER**

According to a study published in the *Journal of Personality and Social Psychology*, when you share a triumph with someone else—like finishing a 5-K or even surviving one killer abs class—and she responds enthusiastically, your perceived value of that event increases and you may become more invested in it. Plus, by sharing workout successes, you're cementing the (perhaps once elusive) idea that exercising is part of your core identity, which can help you stay on that path.

them on logged more exercise hours than people who lacked this support.

## Stage 3 Stalling

Boredom and apathy override your commitment and motivation. You'll use almost anything—work, family, stress, the weather—as an excuse to skip exercise.

**STAY ON TRACK:** Nothing makes motivation evaporate faster than feeling like you're not making any noticeable improvements. The problem: Once women work hard to master a new skill (like holding plank position for 60 seconds or running at a 10-minute-mile pace), they stick with it because, hey, they can do it. But it also impedes progress and breeds big-time boredom. Instead of fixating on a far-off finish line (like losing a certain number of pounds), shift your attention to the instant rewards you can reap from your sweat sessions. (Find five of them starting on the opposite page.)

# BY THE NUMBERS

## 30

Percentage of women who are less active during the winter than when the days are long and the temps are balmy, according to the American College of Sports Medicine.

## Stage 4 Frustration and Surrender

Exercise slides from your list of top priorities. All you want to do is throw in the towel (there's always next month—or year).

**STAY ON TRACK:** Sign a commitment contract. Have you ever bribed yourself with an incentive (like treating yourself to a massage after a month of perfect gym attendance)? Behavioral economists say the flip side—penalties for missing workouts—may be even more effective.

When your drive to sweat is at an all-time low, these types of contracts work by removing and reducing choices. Tapping into your pride can have a powerful effect. Register for a race that requires you to raise donations. You're far less likely to bail if you've already hit up your friends and coworkers to donate. Still not working? Put money on the line. Experts say people will work twice as hard when money is at stake compared with relying only on willpower. Make a friendly wager among coworkers or friends: Everyone ponies up $20 and whoever logs the most workout sessions over 3 months wins the pot.

# 5 Instant Workout Results

▶ Losing sight of your ultimate goals may actually be the real secret to staying motivated: Researchers recently reported that women who tracked instant results after a workout—like feeling happier, more energetic, and less anxious—exercised 34 percent more over the course of a year than those who focused on weight-loss or appearance goals. It makes sense: Physical changes can take weeks and months, which can make working out feel like just another chore.

And that's important, because when it comes to managing a hectic schedule, daily to-dos that don't have tangible and immediate payoffs usually fall off your checklist—including exercise. For an activity to feel like it's worth your time, it has to offer something very important to your daily life, otherwise it quickly begins to feel taxing and harder to justify making time for.

So give your cousin's wedding or that smaller dress size a rest for a minute and focus on these five immediate payoffs—they'll help reboot your motivation to break a sweat. Better yet: Pay careful attention to how you feel after your workouts. Are you more self-confident? Are you less stressed? Finding the payoffs that are most important to you will ensure that you prioritize exercise in your daily routine.

## 1. Get Ahead at Work

Vying for a promotion? Don't sacrifice gym time for late nights at work. Researchers found that women who exercise at least twice a week feel more in control of their jobs and find them less demanding than those who don't work out. According to a survey in the *International Journal of Workplace Health Management*, workers who exercised reported a 32 percent increase in motivation and a 28 percent increase in time management compared to the days they didn't work out.

## 2. Think Sharper

According to a study published in *Clinical Neurophysiology*, 20 minutes of moderate exercise immediately increases attention and cognitive ability. There's a shift in brain activity that enhances executive functioning, which plans, schedules, and coordinates thoughts and actions, explain study authors. This amplified focus can last up to an hour, so schedule a quick workout during a time of day when you tend to be most distracted, or before a time when you'll really need to be on point.

## 3. Get Glowing Skin

A pricey facial is one way to score a better complexion; a single sweat session is another. As your heart rate rises, the increase in blood flow circulates to the surface of your skin, giving you that revitalizing flush of color. Turns out, sweating is good for your skin, too: Some of the water evaporates to cool the body, and the rest is reabsorbed into the skin, giving it a nicely hydrated look post-workout.

## 4. Have Hotter Sex

A study published in the *Journal of Sexual Medicine* found that women who completed a 20-minute treadmill run before watching an erotic film clocked a 150 percent increase in arousal. To take advantage of this, you might want to exercise at home—study authors say the swell in arousal only lasts up to 30 minutes.

 **SLIM-DOWN SECRET**

Don't wait to shed a few pounds before loving your looks. In a study at the Technical University of Lisbon in Portugal, women who were counseled to improve their body image lost a higher percentage of weight than those who weren't. Poor body image can lead to emotional eating and anxiety, which sabotage weight loss. So focus on what you like about your body rather than what you would change.

## 5. Sleep Better

Working out zaps stress and anxiety, and helps your body regulate its own temperature—a trifecta for helping you catch more restful shut-eye. According to a study published in the journal *Mental Health and Physical Activity*, participants who engaged in moderately intense exercise for a total of 150 minutes a week (that's 30 minutes a day, 5 days a week) were able to fall asleep faster and felt less tired during daylight hours. Study authors noted it doesn't matter what time of day you choose to fit in a sweat session, either: Only limited research suggests that late-night physical activity hurts the quality of your sleep.

# Decode Your Exercise Aches and Pains

🢒 Some soreness is to be expected with exercise—especially for beginners or people kicking up their intensity—but you don't need to take the whole "no pain, no gain" mantra so literally. Women runners, for example, tend to push through pain more than men, which leads to injuries that could have been prevented, says Jordan Metzl, MD, sports medicine specialist at the Hospital for Special Surgery in New York City and author of *The Athlete's Book of Home Remedies*. That's not being tough—frankly, it's stupid. Nothing will stop you short of your goals quicker than being sidelined with an injury. Luckily, the most common exercise aches and pains can be spotted and treated at home. Use this cheat sheet from Metzl to keep injuries at bay. (Red-flag exceptions: Go see a doctor if you've experienced a sudden trauma like a fall, or if the pain keeps you up at night or lasts longer than 2 weeks.)

## *Where it hurts:* Lower back (or upper butt)

**WHAT IT COULD BE:** Piriformis syndrome (a tight butt muscle) or a herniated disk (some are worse than others). Both injuries put pressure on the sciatic nerve in your back.

**HOW IT HAPPENED:** The jury's out on what causes piriformis syndrome, but a herniated disk is often the result of improper lifting form or sports that involve rotating.

**DIY TREATMENT:** Take an OTC pain reliever, rest when you feel sore, then hit the gym: One study found that non-weight-bearing exercise (such as riding a stationary bike) and core training relieve back pain better than lying in bed.

**SEE THE DOC IF . . .** You also have a fever, leg weakness, or bladder changes. These symptoms may signal an infection or nerve compression.

## *Where it hurts:* **Elbow**

**WHAT IT COULD BE:** Inflammation of the lateral epicondyle tendon (tennis elbow) or the medial epicondyle tendon (golfer's elbow).

**HOW IT HAPPENED:** Swinging a racket or club is the obvious culprit, but any activity that involves the elbow (like softball) can tax its tendons.

**DIY TREATMENT:** Swallow an OTC pain reliever, ice your elbow, pick up a brace at your local pharmacy to stabilize the tendons, and ease yourself back on course (or court).

 **2-SECOND LIFE CHANGER**

A rosy outlook could mean fewer exercise injuries: Experts found that athletes with an optimistic disposition were less likely to be sidelined with a strain, tear, or other ache over a 2-year period than those who were less optimistic. Try a few of happy people's healthy habits, which are most likely the key to their low injury rates: Ease into new workouts, sleep well, and eat right. If you do get injured, focus on the positive; concentrate on the goal of getting better, say study authors.

**SEE THE DOC IF . . .** You have trouble moving your elbow normally or rotating your palm up and down, or if you have severe swelling and bruising at the joint.

## *Where it hurts:* **Knee**

**WHAT IT COULD BE:** Pain on the outside of the knee signals an inflamed or tight iliotibial band (IT band), the tissue that runs from hip to knee. Pain around the kneecap could be runner's knee—a wearing away of the cartilage under the kneecap.

**HOW IT HAPPENED:** Increasing distance or speed too suddenly is the most common cause of an IT band injury, but research suggests it's also associated with weak hip abductors and glutes. Runner's knee is the result of overtraining, improper running form, or weak quads and hip muscles.

**DIY TREATMENT:** Loosen your IT band with this move: Lie on your side and support your weight with your forearm. Slip a foam roller under your hip and slowly roll down from hip to knee. Repeat this a few times a week. For runner's knee, reduce your mileage to a point that doesn't cause pain, and do leg lifts and presses to strengthen your quads and hamstrings.

**SEE THE DOC IF . . .** Your knee is very swollen or gives out. These signs point to a tear of the anterior cruciate ligament (ACL) or meniscus (knee cartilage).

## *Where it hurts:* **Heel**

**WHAT IT COULD BE:** Plantar fasciitis—inflammation of the connective tissue at the bottom of the foot, which helps support your arch.

**HOW IT HAPPENED:** The usual suspects include overtraining, running on hard surfaces, and wearing worn-out running shoes.

**DIY TREATMENT:** OTC gel heel inserts may help reduce pain and swelling, and street runners may feel relief by switching to a treadmill or trail.

**SEE THE DOC IF . . .** You have severe pain directly after an injury, or if you're unable to rise up on your toes or walk normally.

## *Where it hurts:* **Shin**

**WHAT IT COULD BE:** Medial tibial stress syndrome (better known as shin splints).

**HOW IT HAPPENED:** The "terrible too's" (too much, too soon, too often, too fast, too hard) are usually to blame.

**DIY TREATMENT:** Switch to a non-weight-bearing exercise like swimming or biking for 2 weeks, and ice the area for 20 minutes after each session.

**SEE THE DOC IF . . .** Pain is localized on the outer edge of the shinbone. You may have a stress fracture.

## *Where it hurts:* **Ankle**

**WHAT IT COULD BE:** A sprain, which happens when the ligaments are stretched beyond normal range.

**HOW IT HAPPENED:** You rolled your ankle while playing tennis or soccer, or stepped in a pothole.

**DIY TREATMENT:** Do the RICE method: Rest; ice for 20 minutes three times a day; compress with an elastic bandage; and elevate your foot above heart level as much as possible for 48 hours.

**SEE THE DOC IF . . .** You can't put any weight on the injured foot, or if it's still swollen and painful after 3 days.

*"Impatience never commanded success."*

—EDWIN H. CHAPIN

# Outsmart Fitness Roadblocks

➤ There are dozens of possible reasons your fitness routine took a slide—maybe your work has been too crazy, you moved to a new city, or you were just feeling under the weather. It's never just about the physical roadblock; there are logistical and psychological challenges, as well. No matter where you are now, use these strategies to pave the way to a hotter, healthier body.

## You Work Insane Hours

*Twelve-hour workdays don't leave much time for boot camps or long runs in the park (or even short runs in the park!).*

**TRAINING TIP:** Plan workouts when you have the fewest conflicts, which for most people is first thing in the a.m. Not an early riser? Inch your alarm back a little every few days; it will gradually reset your body's clock, so you'll have more energy. Eventually, you'll be waking up a half hour early no problem—plenty of time to fit in any workout from Part II. If you love (or need) to hit the gym at night, get changed before you leave work. Otherwise, it can be tempting to head straight home—or catch the tail end of happy hour.

**MENTAL TRICK:** Keep this in mind: Not only can daily exercise help your mental sharpness, learning, and memory, but a recent study found that working out three or more times a week leads to higher pay.

## You're in the New-Love Bubble

*Morning exercisers find it tough to get out of bed when there's a guy lying next to them; evening exercisers have a hard time passing up romantic dinners in favor of workouts.*

**TRAINING TIP:** Work out when he's not around—say, during your lunch break or girls' night (hit up a Pilates class and then head to dinner). Even better, get him to do it with you. It's amazing how simply working out together can improve communication, strengthen mutual support, and give you more shared interests.

**MENTAL TRICK:** Turns out, exercise can do more to boost your sex life than sharing a bottle of wine: Research shows that frequent exercisers have more feelings of being sexually desirable. And, yes, spending time with your man is important, but one study found that women who do their own thing have happier marriages.

## You Were Sidelined by Injury

*People either rush into their former workouts, which puts them at risk for another injury, or are so afraid of getting hurt again that they put it off altogether.*

**TRAINING TIP:** After your doctor clears you, scale back your routine by at least 50 percent for 2 weeks. Back off a bit if you begin nursing the area or feel an uptick in acute pain, which can ultimately throw off your form and cause new injuries.

**MENTAL TRICK:** Challenge those negative, "poor me" thoughts. Staying positive may sound like psychobabble, but it really works. And while it's normal to be nervous, it's important to trust your doctor's orders when he gives you the A-OK.

## Your Social Calendar Has Cramped Your Gym Time

*Weeks of eating, drinking, and partying (and not exercising) have left you feeling overwhelmed by the idea of having to undo the damage.*

**TRAINING TIP:** Hitting the gym hard can quickly lead to burnout. Rather than double your sessions or hours of cardio, choose manageable activities, like yoga or short strength circuits.

**MENTAL TRICK:** There's this feeling of, "Oh, what the hell, it's too late now." But keep in mind, it's easier to drop 2 pounds than 10, which could happen if you delay your comeback. You don't have to give up all indulgences cold turkey, either. Make one healthy swap or change each day to ease back on track.

## You Just Made a Big Move

*Between hunting for new digs and packing up your life, your running shoes may have gotten buried in the boxes.*

Scope out your fitness options before you pack the moving van. If you join the local gym or ID new running routes prior to your move, you'll have a workout plan ready once your stuff is unpacked. It maintains your commitment to regular exercise—regardless of geography. To find running routes in your new neighborhood, go to usatf.org/routes.

## You Just Had a Baby

*Intense exercise is usually off-limits for 6 weeks postpartum. After that, sheer exhaustion can keep moms couched.*

**TRAINING TIP:** Even if you're wiped, pop in a DVD or slip your baby in the stroller for a brisk walk. It will boost your energy and help you sleep better. And, in the long term, exercising will fend off postpartum depression.

**MENTAL TRICK:** Women can become obsessed with dropping the baby weight and get frustrated if it doesn't happen right away. After all, we see celebs on the red carpet weeks after popping out an offspring looking svelte as ever—it can't be all thanks to Spanx. But all that does is add stress, which is basically salt on the wound. (You'll hear more about how stress stalls your weight-loss efforts in Chapter 9.) Make your goal more realistic, though, and you'll be more likely to tackle it: Mentally commit to just 5 to 10 minutes of exercise. If you don't feel energized after that time period has elapsed, try again later or take the day off and try again tomorrow.

*"The difference between a successful person and others is not a lack of strength, not a lack of knowledge, but rather a lack in will."*

—VINCE LOMBARDI

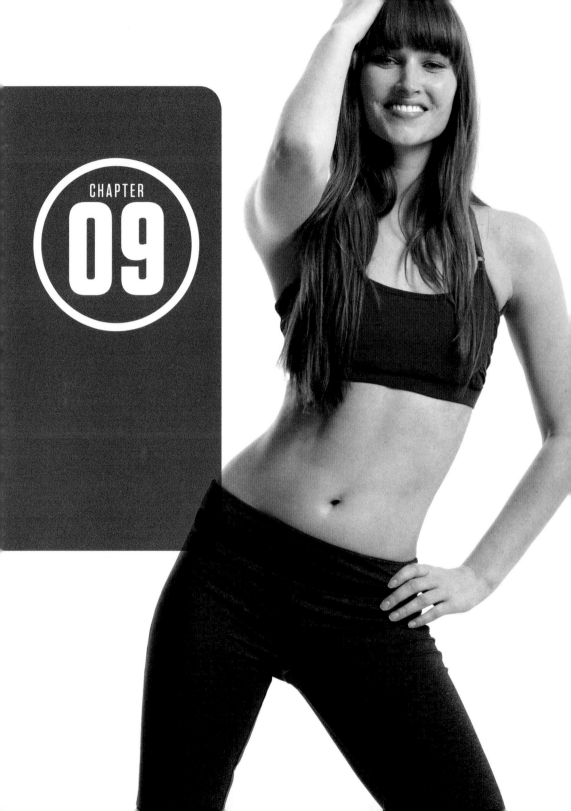

CHAPTER

09

# A Better Body—No Sweat!

*6 secrets to looking slimmer instantly*

**W**hile the majority of this book focuses on better eating and exercise habits, there's another piece of the puzzle you're likely neglecting: To speed your results, research shows that what you do when you're not exercising is nearly as important as the workout itself (if not more important).

Before you roll your eyes and think, *"Oh, great, one more thing to add to my already maxed out to-do list,"* hear me out. Exercise is literally a process of breaking down your muscle fibers, creating tiny microscopic tears; as soon as you slip off your sneakers after a workout, your body starts repairing that "damage" to your muscles. In fact, it's this recovery process—not the actual workout itself—that makes you stronger and leaner.

But it goes far beyond just crashing on the couch after a tough workout. Overlook the minimum-effort moves in this chapter and you could be stalling your progress. Follow these six secrets to use your downtime to increase energy, boost metabolism, reduce soreness, and drop weight faster. Trust me, when it comes to shortcuts, these are *not* the places to take them.

## *"How you do anything is how you do everything."*

—TOM DAVIN

## NO-SWEAT SECRET #1:

# Sneak in More Shut-Eye

I know, I know—if you dropped a pound every time you heard about the advantages of sleep, you'd never have to work out again. I truly realize and value its importance, and yet I'm still guilty of logging way too many nights at far fewer than the standard 8-hour recommendation. But even if you think you operate just fine on less-than-average hours (like I do), prioritizing shut-eye truly may be one of the best things you can do to meet your body-shaping goals.

For starters, sleep increases production of tissue-repairing growth hormones, meaning you'll score some of the best muscle recovery under the covers. When Stanford University researchers had 1,000 volunteers report the number of hours they slept each night, they found the participants who got less than 8 hours of sleep per night had higher body fat content. It's a weight-gain double whammy: Lack of sleep prompts your body to consume more calories and shut down its ability to recognize a full stomach. When you're tired, your gut produces more ghrelin, a chemical that triggers sugar cravings. Meanwhile, fatigue suppresses leptin, a fat-cell hormone that tells your brain, "Okay, stop eating now." Then, there's the possibly larger issue: When you're awake more hours of the day, you have more opportunities to eat.

Your sweet spot: somewhere between 6 to 8 hours a night. A study found that people who snoozed for fewer than 6 were more likely

 **2-SECOND LIFE CHANGER**

Set your alarm for an hour before bed, then power down: Not only are electronics distracting, but the type of light they emit can affect your sleep quality.

## 2-SECOND LIFE CHANGER

A study conducted by researchers at the University of Colorado Sleep and Chronobiology Laboratory found that people who were limited to just 5 hours of sleep over the course of 5 days gained, on average, nearly 2 pounds. But there are two slightly more subtle points of the study that are worth highlighting: All the participants had access to unlimited amounts of food, and they also weren't told to try to watch their intake. You can fend off the reported weight gain by tackling both: Keep high-calorie snacks and treats out of the house, and your weekly and long-term goals in plain sight (try writing them down and sticking them on the fridge).

to suffer a stroke or heart attack, and those who got more than 8 were also more likely to have heart woes. Too little sleep is associated with higher levels of stress hormones, while too much time between the sheets may indicate an underlying condition like depression.

Hey, even I see those numbers and shake my head. There are going to be nights where even 6 hours is tough to squeeze in. So remember this: Sleep quality is just as important as the total number of hours you're under the covers. Things like caffeine, alcohol, and late-night TV can keep you from feeling reenergized when the alarm goes off. So, especially on nights you may be skimping, keep an eye on those things to ensure you're getting the best quality of sleep—no matter how many hours you manage to fit in.

## Motivate No Matter What

One question I hear from a lot of women is, "Should I exercise in the morning even if I'm dead tired?" I know the feeling, because I struggle with it all the time. If you truly didn't get enough shut-eye (you rolled in at 3 a.m. or were up all night with a crying baby), crawl back under the covers. Research has found that when dieters were sleep deprived they lost less body fat and more lean muscle mass than when they tallied more Zs. What's more, exercising when you're too drained can take your focus off proper form, upping your risk of injury.

If you're just feeling groggy, get your butt out of bed, but give yourself an out. Commit to do half of your workout—or even one set of it. Knowing that you can cut it short will get you out the door, which is the hardest part. (On a few super-sleepy mornings, I have served up this compromise: I have to get to the gym, but if I'm still not feeling it when I get there, I can just shower and get ready for work.) Chances are, you'll pick up steam as you go and feel energized enough to finish. (I've never actually taken my shower-only shortcut.)

# NIGHT LIGHT

If you love to read on your tablet, know this: A study in *Applied Ergonomics* found that using a tablet for 2 hours suppresses melatonin production—a hormone necessary for sleep—by 23 percent. Here's how to get in a chapter before bed and a full night of Zs:

✓ Limit yourself to 1 hour and turn off other lights in the room.
✓ Invest in a filter that blocks shortwave blue-light emissions.
✓ Set your tablet to display large white text on top of black.

## NO-SWEAT SECRET #2:

# Stop Stressing

 Your daily commute. Your in-laws. Your bank statement. Your never-ending to-do list. I hear you—life is hard. But when you get all bent out of shape about any of these daily stressors, it's not just your mood that takes a hit. Your body has a physical reaction, as well.

That headache-inducing, anxiety-producing feeling is your body's way of trying to maintain balance in the midst of the madness, which it deals with in the only way it knows how: by signaling the adrenal glands to release the stress hormones cortisol and adrenaline (the docs call it epinephrine).

## ⏱ 2-SECOND LIFE CHANGER

When tension runs high, we reach for fattening foods. To keep your hand out of the office candy jar, keep it far, far away. In one study, participants who had to walk 6 feet to reach candy ate up to seven fewer chocolates per day than when the jar was conveniently located at their desk.

You may be more familiar with adrenaline as the fight-or-flight hormone; it gives you instant energy, so you can get out of (what your body perceives as) harm's way. But then there's cortisol, which after it's released by your adrenal glands may interfere with the signals that control appetite (ghrelin) and satiety (leptin), research suggests. As if that's not bad enough, cortisol inhibits the muscle-repair process and alters your metabolism, so that your body stores more calories as fat instead of burning them off. Even worse, that fat tends to settle around your waistline, because visceral fat—or intra-abdominal fat, which resides underneath the abdominal muscles—has more cortisol receptors than fat below the skin.

> *"Life is 10 percent
> what happens to you
> and 90 percent
> how you react to it."*
>
> —CHARLES R. SWINDOLL

# 6 Simple Stress Busters

You don't have to resign yourself to feeling frazzled. What distinguishes one person's meltdown from another's composure is their perception of control over the situation. Try these strategies to shrug off any tough situation in a flash.

## 1. TEA OFF

In a study at University College in London, volunteers drank the equivalent of a cup of black tea before completing two stressful tasks. Afterward, their cortisol levels dropped an average of 47 percent, compared with 27 percent for the people who didn't imbibe.

## 2. JUST SAY "%&* IT!"

Swearing reduces stress, according to research published in the *Leadership & Organization Development Journal*. Now, I'm not saying that gives you a pass to drop F-bombs in the middle of your office, but a strategically placed expletive in the privacy of your car, kitchen, or bedroom can help you blow off steam.

### 3. PRESS THE ISSUE

Acupressure is a quick and effective tension reliever—it can reduce stress by up to 39 percent, according to researchers at Hong Kong Polytechnic University. For fast relief, massage the fleshy area between your thumb and index finger for 20 to 30 seconds.

### 4. TREAT YOURSELF

Flavonoids in cocoa relax your body's blood vessels so that arteries can dilate, reducing blood pressure, found a study published in the *Proceedings of the National Academy of Sciences*. Look for dark chocolate or cocoa powder, which have more of the stress-busting compound than milk chocolate, and keep it to one serving.

### 5. TAKE A YOUTUBE TIME-OUT

Just the anticipation of laughing significantly decreases levels of the stress hormones DOPAC, cortisol, and epinephrine, according to researchers at Loma Linda University in California.

### 6. CHEW THE FAT

According to a study from the University of Pittsburgh, people with the highest blood levels of EPA and DHA omega-3 fatty acids are happier, less impulsive, and generally more agreeable. Boost your mood by adding foods rich in omega-3s—salmon, herring, and sardines top the list. Or try a daily supplement of 400 milligrams each of EPA and DHA fish oils.

*"Every day do something that will inch you closer to a better tomorrow."*

—DOUG FIREBAUGH

## NO-SWEAT SECRET #3:

# Drink Up

Water may very well be one of the most undervalued nutrients. Proper hydration improves exercise performance, lubricates your joints, and even keeps your

## 2-SECOND LIFE CHANGER

Eight glasses a day (or 64 ounces) may be the go-to rule for water consumption, but experts advise downing an additional 16 to 20 ounces for every hour you train. Sound like way too much? Remember, most standard bottles of water contain 16 ounces, so four of them (not eight) is what you're shooting for.

skin healthy and glowing. It's also critical to dropping weight—so even if you're killing it at the gym, you could be negating the calorie-burning advantages if you aren't drinking enough $H_2O$. Turns out, well-hydrated cells may actually boost your metabolism: After women upped their $H_2O$ consumption to 1 liter a day for a year, 5 pounds of their weight loss was credited to the water.

What's more, dehydration (even when it's mild) can take a toll on your mood, reports the *Journal of Nutrition*. When researchers had study participants walk on a treadmill for 40 minutes, they found that losing as little as 1 percent of body weight in fluid led to decreases in mood, concentration, memory, and energy.

And before you reach for that snack because you're "hungry," pause and

## # BY THE NUMBERS

**17** Percentage more reps people could do in three sets when they were well hydrated, according to researchers at the University of Connecticut.

drink a glass of water: If you've been eating regularly, it's likely a sign that you're thirsty.

# Get Moving

➤ You may feel like rewarding yourself with some downtime, but doing a low-key activity the day after a big workout will prolong the muscle-sculpting perks of increased circulation. Fresh bloodflow brings fresh nutrients to your muscles and helps flush waste products. What's more, staying active has also been proven to reduce post-exercise muscle soreness and suppress nervous-system activity that can result in poor sleep.

Take a restorative yoga class or go on a walk with friends at a conversational pace. If you're sitting behind a desk all day, stroll around the office for about 10 minutes every couple of hours to get things moving. Then, prepare for a different kind of reward: a less-painful gym session tomorrow.

# Massage Your Muscles

➤ A post-workout massage isn't just an indulgence—research shows that it boosts strength recovery by 60 percent, and it may be one of the most effective strategies to prevent pain and injury.

Remember those tiny microscopic tears in the muscle fibers

caused by your workouts? As they repair and try to heal themselves, patches of scar tissue can form—those "knots" in your muscles that hurt like hell. For the muscle to regain maximum strength and flexibility, the scar tissue needs to become aligned and integrated with the muscle fibers. That's where massage comes in: It reduces inflammation in the tissue and increases blood flow to the area—two things that speed up recovery and help "smooth out" any kinks.

The hands-on approach helps another part of your body that you may not know about. When your muscles are chronically tight, the surrounding fascia tightens along with them. Never heard of fascia? It's a cobweblike casing of connective tissue that surrounds every muscle, tendon, ligament, nerve, and bone in your body; it keeps each internal body part separate and allows it to slide easily with your movements. To experts like Todd Durkin (you should read everything he writes on this topic and every topic), fascia quality plays a critical role in performance, joint stability, injury, and chronic pain—and it's something we don't pay nearly enough attention to.

In its healthy state, fascia is smooth and supple and slides easily, allowing you to move and stretch in every direction at a full range of motion. But it's not just like plastic wrap; fascia reacts to stress and can tighten—as it does in response to repetitive motions, trauma and injury, or even poor posture—and, over time, the fascia becomes rigid, compressing the muscles and nerves it surrounds. Sticky adhesions form between fascial surfaces, and they can be tough to eliminate. Unfortunately, our bodies don't have a natural mechanism for getting rid of them.

By correcting (aligning and smoothing out) areas of scar tissue and other muscular irregularities, massage and self-massage techniques break the muscular pain cycle at its root, accelerate healing, and restore muscular balance.

Using a foam roller on your fascia is different than on your muscles. Fascia works in slower cycles than muscles, both contracting and stretching more slowly. Be gentle and slow in your movements, and when you find an area of tension, hold sustained pressure for 3 to 5 minutes. Practice self-massage with the same rules.

## NO-SWEAT SECRET #6:
# Straighten Up

▶ Your mom may have told you that slouching was merely poor manners, but poor posture can actually prevent you from getting the body you're after, despite any amount of exercise. (I bet that got you to sit up straight.)

That's because over time, poor posture takes a serious toll on your spine, shoulders, hips, and knees. In fact, it can cause a cascade of structural flaws throughout your body that lead to back and joint pain, reduced flexibility, and compromised muscles—all of which limit your ability to burn fat and build strength.

Poor posture could also be to blame if you're prone to side stitches during workouts. Research in the *Journal of Science and Medicine in*

# POSTURE PROBLEMS—SOLVED!

Sure, hunched shoulders are easy to spot, but not all postural issues are as easy to pinpoint. Wear something form fitting and have someone snap two full-body photos of you—one from the front and one from the side. Relax your muscles and stand as tall as you can, feet hip-width apart. Use the exercises in "Lean and Tall in Minutes" on page 256 to improve any problems you uncover.

## FROM THE FRONT . . .

1. Look at your shoulders. One shouldn't appear higher than the other.

2. Check out your kneecaps. Do they point inward, causing your knees to nearly touch when your legs are straight?

3. Do your toes point outward more than 10 degrees? This means you're duck-footed.

## FROM THE SIDE . . .

1. If your ear is in front of the midpoint of your shoulder, your head is too far forward.

2. Can you see your shoulder blades? This means your back is rounded.

3. If your lower spine is arched significantly and your hips tilt forward (you may have a belly pooch, even if you don't have an ounce of fat on your body), this means you have an anterior pelvic tilt.

*Sport* found that people who round their upper backs are more prone to these crippling cramps and feel more intense discomfort. The reason: A hunched posture may compress the nerves that run along your spine and into your belly, making them more sensitive to pain.

# Lean and Tall in Minutes

Stand taller (and look 10 pounds lighter!) with these simple fixes from Bill Hartman, PT, CSCS, co-owner of Indianapolis Fitness and Sports Training.

### 1. FORWARD HEAD

**THE PROBLEM:** Stiff muscles in the back of your neck.

**THE FIX:** Moving only your head, drop your chin down and in toward your sternum while stretching the back of your neck. Hold for a count of 5; do this 10 times a day.

### 2. ROUNDED SHOULDERS

**THE PROBLEM:** Weakness in the middle and lower parts of your trapezius (the large muscle that spans your shoulders and back).

**THE FIX:** Lie facedown with your arms overhead in a *Y* position on the floor. Squeeze your shoulder blades together and raise your arms a few inches off the floor; hold for 2 or 3 seconds, then return to the start. Do two sets of 12 reps.

*Quick tip: Rounded shoulders compress your ribs and abdomen, making your torso appear wider than it actually is.*

### 3. ANTERIOR PELVIC TILT

**THE PROBLEM:** Tight hip flexors.

**THE FIX:** Kneel on your left knee, with your right foot on the floor in front of you, knee bent. Press forward until you feel the stretch in your left hip. Tighten your butt muscles on your left side until you feel the front of your hip stretching comfortably. Reach upward with your left arm and stretch to the right side. Hold for a count of 30 seconds. That's 1 rep; do 3 on each side.

## 4. ELEVATED SHOULDER

**THE PROBLEM:** The muscle under your chest (running from your ribs to your shoulder blades) is weak.

**THE FIX:** Sit upright in a chair with your hands next to your hips, palms down on the seat, arms

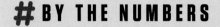

# BY THE NUMBERS

## 34

Percentage of women ages 18 and older who suffer from chronic hurt, reports the *Journal of Pain*.

straight. Without moving your arms, push down on the chair until your hips lift up off the seat and your torso rises. Hold for 5 seconds. That's 1 rep; do two or three sets of 12 reps daily.

## 5. PIGEON TOES

**THE PROBLEM:** Weak glutes (butt muscles).

**THE FIX:** Lie on one side with your knees bent 90 degrees and your heels together. Keeping your hips still, raise your top knee upward, separating your knees like a clamshell. Pause for 5 seconds, then lower your knee to the starting position. That's 1 rep. Perform two or three sets of 12 reps on each side daily.

## 6. DUCK FEET

**THE PROBLEM:** Your oblique muscles and hip flexors are weak.

**THE FIX:** Get into a pushup position with your feet resting on a stability ball. Without rounding your lower back, tuck your knees under your torso, using your feet to roll the ball toward your body, then back to the starting position. That's 1 rep. Do two or three sets of 6 to 12 reps daily.

# Improve Your Posture—All Day Long!

Proper form isn't only important during your workouts. There are endless situations throughout the day that can hurt your posture—and we hardly give them thought. Here's the best, and safest, way to . . .

### PICK UP A TODDLER

Bend your knees—so as not to strain your hips, spine, or neck—and crouch all the way down at eye level with the child. Pull the munchkin close to your body—as in a hug—and slowly stand straight up.

### STAND AT A COCKTAIL PARTY

Keep your knees slightly bent and your weight over your entire foot. High heels shift your weight forward, so consciously think about having your weight in the heel. Change your stance every few minutes.

### DRIVE A CAR

With your neck and shoulders relaxed, lightly grip the steering wheel at 10:00 and 2:00 à la your driving-school days. Move your eyes independently of your head—there's no need for too much neck movement.

### SIT AT YOUR DESK

Center yourself on your sit bones, then think about your spine drawing straight up toward

 **2-SECOND LIFE CHANGER**

Feeling exhausted during or after a tough workout puts people in a familiar position—usually hunched over, hands on their knees, gasping for air. Turns out, this could be making things worse. Rounding your back presses the rib cage and internal organs against your lungs, keeping them from expanding efficiently. The result: Less oxygen gets to your muscles, which makes you run and recover more slowly. Instead, stand tall and place your hands behind your head (elbows out) or stretch them overhead during rest breaks.

the ceiling and your shoulders extending outward. Keep your neck long and still, and get up and move every 15 minutes to stay loose.

## 2-SECOND LIFE CHANGER

Need to realign your spine? Gently correct the bend with this stretch: Lie on the floor and place a towel folded to 4 inches thick under your shoulders (perpendicular to your spine); clasp your hands behind your head. Lie on the towel for 30 seconds; sit up for 30 seconds. Repeat three times.

## WASH DISHES

To reach into an overflowing sink full of dishes, hinge forward from your hips (like you're sticking your butt out to close a car door behind you), rather than hunching down with your shoulders or upper back. Move your head, neck, and torso as a single unit, so that your spine stays long.

*"The greatest results in life are usually attained by simple means and the exercise of ordinary qualities. These may for the most part be summed in these two: common sense and perseverance."*

—OWEN FELTHAM

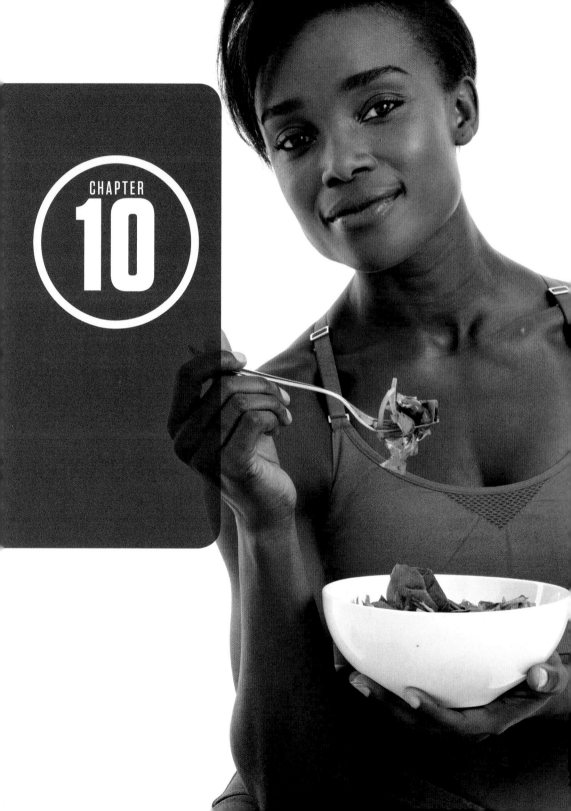

CHAPTER

# 10

# Meal Makeovers

*Delicious, healthy, and quick solutions to eating a little better every day*

**W**hy and how women eat usually boils down to three things—time, money, and health. Unfortunately, the first two are often the most persuasive, and you feel forced to make a trade-off: Whip up easy grub that isn't kind to your waistline, or spend the entire night preparing delicious, nutritious fare.

There are a lot of preconceived notions about healthy eating: It's boring, it's time consuming, it's expensive. In a recent study, 41 percent of women cited "not enough time" as the reason they don't eat better. And when researchers at the University of Minnesota School of Public Health surveyed 530 adults about their attitudes toward fast foods, they found that people already know fast food is unhealthy (not a shocker), but the primary reasons they purchased it anyway were perceived convenience and a dislike for cooking.

Well, not anymore. In this chapter, you won't find set-in-stone meal plans or elaborate recipes. Instead, you'll find approachable, affordable ingredients combined in a straightforward, easy-to-follow way. You'll learn basic, quick tips that can help you improve your food options—whether they're coming from your kitchen, the grocery store, or the drive-thru—to make your current diet, whatever it is, better.

This means you won't have to do a grand, unmanageable overhaul. You'll always be a cereal-in-the-morning person despite people telling you over and over about the perks of protein? Nothing could make you reconsider your twice-a-week takeout? That's totally fine—you'll find ways to keep nonnegotiables in your diet, but just make them a little better. You don't have to institute every single change right away, or do them every day, to get a better body. Your goal: Make just *one* meal better today. Or make a few smart swaps throughout the day—replacing a slice of cheese with a handful of spinach to cut 100 calories from your omelet, or cutting about 77 calories per ounce by dressing your salad with lemon juice rather than balsamic vinaigrette.

That's progress. That's one step closer to the body of your dreams.

# Breakfast Essentials

➤ You've heard it a thousand times: Breakfast is one of the most important meals of the day. And the heartier your first meal is, the better. In one study published in the *American Journal of Epidemiology,* volunteers who got 22 to 55 percent of their total calories at breakfast gained only 1.7 pounds, on average, over 4 years. Those who ate zero to 11 percent of their calories in the morning gained nearly 3 pounds. Lucky for you, it doesn't have to be time consuming or complicated. Fire up your metabolism and control hunger and cravings all day long with these simple strategies to boost your breakfast.

## Start a Cereal Smackdown

Pouring yourself a bowl of cereal can jump-start your day (research shows that people who do so also consume more produce and whole grains during the day). But in some cases, it can derail your diet. Satisfy the morning munchies without packing on pounds.

### WATCH THE LABEL

Choose cereals that have at least 3 grams of fiber (it's good for weight loss and health, and it will keep you fuller longer), fewer than 200 calories per serving, and no more than 8 grams of sugar.

### TRY NEW GRAINS

You don't have to look for just whole grains, such as whole wheat and whole oats, in the ingredient list, anymore. Many cereals, such as those in the Sunrise line by Nature's Path, have lesser-known yet tasty whole grains like quinoa, buckwheat, and amaranth.

## PREVENT OVERPOURING

Resist filling your bowl to the brim. Serving sizes vary between cereals (for example, a serving of plain Cheerios is 1 cup, while Honey Nut Cheerios is ¾ cup), and our serving bowls are often much larger than we realize. Get an accurate visual reference by measuring out one serving into your bowl the first time you eat the cereal.

## DOWNSIZE DINING

Eat cereal out of a coffee mug to trick your mind into thinking you're eating more. Some experts also recommend eating with a smaller spoon, which they say can slow you down.

## GO SPLITS

Can't give up your sugary cereal? Slowly dial back by adding a percentage of a healthier pick. So, instead of having 1 cup, mix in ½ cup of a healthier option (like Fiber One).

# Discover Milk without the Moo

While cow's milk contains nutrients such as calcium, vitamin D, and protein, people are turning to nondairy varieties because of allergies, lactose intolerance, and concerns about hormones and antibiotics. Not all faux milks are created nutritionally or calorically equal, so consult this guide before you drink up.

## ALMOND MILK

The least caloric of the bunch, it's fortified with vitamin E, a powerful antioxidant that fights ultraviolet damage, as well as calcium and vitamins A and D. But while almonds themselves are a good source of fiber and protein, the milk contains skimpy amounts of these nutrients (because the milk is made by grinding the nuts and mixing them with water).

**TASTE:** Creamy, rich, and slightly nutty with a hint of sweetness.

**BEST IN:** Smoothies, coffee, and cereal.

## COCONUT MILK

It has the least amount of sodium and can be fairly low-cal—even some flavored kinds will cost you only 90 calories per serving. Plus, most brands are fortified with half a day's worth of vitamin $B_{12}$, a brain-boosting nutrient. The majority of fat is saturated, but at 5 grams per serving, it constitutes less than 8 percent of your total daily value for fat.

**TASTE:** Thick, creamy, and, yep, coconut-y.

**BEST IN:** Coffee, tea, pudding, smoothies, and oatmeal—it's a go-to thickener.

## SOY MILK

It has almost as much protein as cow's milk, plus plant chemicals that may help inhibit absorption of cholesterol. It's often fortified, so shake

### SLIM-DOWN SECRET

Dairy gets all the credit for fortifying your frame, but there may be another food that can help you bone up: olive oil. In a study published in the *Journal of Clinical Endocrinology and Metabolism*, people who consumed a Mediterranean diet plus virgin olive oil for 2 years saw an increase in osteo-calcin, a protein that's a marker of bone growth. Those who didn't up their oil intake experienced no such change.

the carton well—added calcium tends to settle at the bottom.

**TASTE:** Faintly sweet. Some varieties have a slight tofu flavor.

**BEST IN:** Creamy soups, salad dressings, sauces, casseroles, and other savory dishes. Vanilla-flavored varieties are great in coffee or tea (or by the glass!).

## RICE MILK

The drink's carb content is a double-edged sword: Having a glass before or after a workout will give you fuel (and fluid to hydrate), but if you're trying to drop a few pounds, it's best to eat whole grain carbs, which contain filling fiber (rice milk has zero).

**TASTE:** Light, watery, and sweet.

**BEST IN:** Desserts, baked goods, pancakes, and French toast. Its natural sweetness complements indulgent foods; use it to reduce a recipe's sugar content.

# The Incredible Egg

Consider it your pound-shedding partner in crime: Researchers from the University of Louisiana found eating eggs for breakfast can cut your daily food intake by up to 415 calories. At less than 80 calories, a single egg is packed with fat-fighting vitamin D and high-quality proteins that keep you feeling full longer. And despite its bad press, if your cholesterol is healthy, you can eat eggs every day.

Use eggs to quickly transform leftovers—vegetables, a hunk of cheese, the last few slices of bread—into a savory frittata. (Just make sure egg-based dishes, such as casseroles or quiches, are cooked to an internal temperature of 160°F or higher by using a food thermometer.)

Eggs will keep in your refrigerator for 3 to 5 weeks. You don't have to worry about pounding through a dozen in a week, either. (Fun fact: Older eggs are actually better for boiling because they're easier to peel.)

### 1

Stir 2 eggs with a fork until the white and yolk are well blended. Add 1 slice Canadian bacon, diced, and chopped tomato and microwave for 2 minutes and 30 seconds or until the eggs are firmly set.

### 2

Heat a cup of spicy, not too chunky salsa in a skillet. Add 2 handfuls of tortilla chips and cook until slightly softened, but retain pockets of crunchiness—about 90 seconds. Top with a fried egg, thinly sliced onion, crumbled cheese, and a squeeze of lime.

### 3

Simmer half a can of black beans with a cup of chicken broth. Crack 2 eggs directly into the mixture and cook until the whites are set. Hit with hot sauce to taste.

## Overhaul Your Oatmeal

Oatmeal's heart-smart, waistline-trimming reputation is so solid, you might not think to check the label. But some brands cram in artificial ingredients and sweeten-

### SLIM-DOWN SECRET

Steel-cut oats are no better for you than rolled or quick oats. Less processing does make steel-cut oats chewier, and it may slightly dampen the effect the carbs have on your blood sugar, but this effect is slight. The real benefit—cholesterol-lowering, heart-protecting, waistline-shrinking beta-glucan fiber—can be found in any bowl.

ers that displace the benefits. A better solution: Ditch the packets and stir up a bowl of plain oats, then boost the flavor and nutrition of your morning meal with these quick recipes.

Each recipe is based on ½ cup dry rolled oats, prepared with water. Or make it with ½ cup fat-free milk for added protein, calcium, and vitamin D, and fewer than 50 extra calories.

(If you're pressed for time, simply stir a spoonful of peanut butter or vanilla protein powder into a bowl of plain instant oatmeal.)

## OATY EGG FLORENTINE

No need to choose between two morning faves. Eggs and oats collide deliciously for an extra-hearty, protein-filled morning meal. Make it: Stir ¼ cup chopped baby spinach into the oatmeal. Top with 1 thin slice of Swiss cheese and 1 large egg, sunny-side up.

PER SERVING: 350 CALORIES, 18 G PROTEIN, 34 G CARBOHYDRATES, 15 G TOTAL FAT, 6 G SATURATED FAT, 5 G FIBER, 140 MG SODIUM

## STRAWBERRIES AND CREAM

No packet comes close to packing the protein, vitamins, antioxidants, and flavor in this combo. Make it: Add ¼ cup plain nonfat Greek yogurt, 1 tablespoon honey, and ¼ cup sliced strawberries to the oatmeal and stir well. Garnish with strawberry halves.

PER SERVING: 300 CALORIES, 12 G PROTEIN, 61 G CARBOHYDRATES, 4 G TOTAL FAT, 0.5 G SATURATED FAT, 6 G FIBER, 25 MG SODIUM

## MAPLE-BACON OATMEAL

You can argue the merits of turkey bacon versus regular, but one thing's for sure: This salty-sweet combination is an instant meal makeover. Make it: Cook 2 slices of turkey bacon. Mix the oatmeal with 2 table-spoons maple syrup, then crumble the bacon on top.

PER SERVING: 360 CALORIES, 11 G PROTEIN, 61 G CARBOHYDRATES, 8 G TOTAL FAT, 2 G SATURATED FAT, 5 G FIBER, 390 MG SODIUM

## CHAI OATMEAL

Give oats a germ-fighting kick with a spice blend that combines stomach-soothing ginger with the antibacterial power of honey. Make it: Mix the oatmeal with a pinch each of ground cardamom, cinnamon, cloves, and ginger and ¼ cup low-fat milk. Drizzle with 1 teaspoon honey and 2 tablespoons slivered almonds.

PER SERVING: 320 CALORIES, 11 G PROTEIN, 47 G CARBOHYDRATES, 11 G TOTAL FAT, 1.5 G SATURATED FAT, 8 G FIBER, 30 MG SODIUM

## CACIO E PEPE

Breakfast takes a savory turn when you prepare oats Roman-style with cheese and black pepper. Make it: Mix the oatmeal with 2 tablespoons shredded pecorino Romano cheese and ½ teaspoon freshly ground black pepper. Top with 2 teaspoons heart-healthy extra-virgin olive oil.

PER SERVING: 330 CALORIES, 11 G PROTEIN, 35 G CARBOHYDRATES, 16 G TOTAL FAT, 4.5 G SATURATED FAT, 6 G FIBER, 250 MG SODIUM

# Slim Down with Yogurt

It's no surprise yogurt was one of the top foods associated with weight loss according to a 20-year study by the Harvard School of Public Health: It's packed with protein and calcium, and the Greek variety has even more—plus, its thick texture is traditionally achieved by straining, which removes not only the liquid whey, but also some of the sugar and salt. Recent research uncovered another benefit of yogurt: Eating about 6 ounces of the low-fat variety three times a week was linked to a 31 percent lower risk of high blood pressure. However, some companies use thickeners to create that consistency, so check the ingredients panel for milk protein concentrate or cornstarch, two common thickeners, or other unfamiliar ingredients.

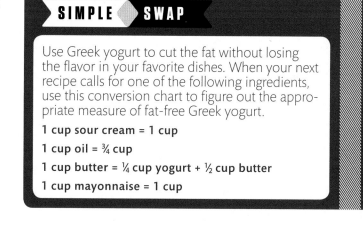

**SIMPLE SWAP**

Use Greek yogurt to cut the fat without losing the flavor in your favorite dishes. When your next recipe calls for one of the following ingredients, use this conversion chart to figure out the appropriate measure of fat-free Greek yogurt.

**1 cup sour cream = 1 cup**

**1 cup oil = ¾ cup**

**1 cup butter = ¼ cup yogurt + ½ cup butter**

**1 cup mayonnaise = 1 cup**

# Blend a Better Smoothie

Assemble the recommended nine servings of fruits and vegetables on your kitchen counter, and the prospect of fitting them into 24 hours may feel next to impossible. Blend them into an ice-cold smoothie, however, and it's suddenly much less daunting. This is just one reason why I don't see this trend going anywhere anytime soon. Smoothies are a super-simple—not to mention, portable and delicious—way to get more fruits and vegetables (yes, vegetables!) into your daily diet. Use these rules to add power, protein, and personality to your own smoothies.

 **2-SECOND LIFE CHANGER**

Layer your ingredients in the right order for a better blend. Pour in liquids first, then watery fruits (think grapes and watermelon), soft fruits and vegetables (like bananas and avocados), hard fruits and vegetables (such as carrots and celery), and greens, then add ice to the top.

## RESPECT THE RATIO

For every 3 cups of produce, you'll need about 1 cup of liquid. Once you learn the basic proportions of solids to liquids, you can toss almost anything into your smoothie.

## OPT FOR LOW FAT

When choosing your dairy or dairy-free ingredients like milk, almond milk, and yogurt, the less fat, the better. Once blended, you can't tell the difference between full fat and fat free. And skip flavored yogurts—flavors add extra sugar that you don't need.

## SKIP THE RAW EGGS

They're not worth the salmonella risk. Use other sources to add protein, such as protein powder, tofu, cottage cheese, or peanut butter.

# BETTER THAN THE BAKERY: MAKE THESE BLUEBERRY-YOGURT MUFFINS

**Coffee shop baked goods are** delicious and convenient, but they are often oversized and loaded with sugar, refined white flour, and saturated fat. By swapping out the usual ingredients for things like yogurt and whole wheat flour—not to mention, adding hunger-squashing wheat germ—these muffins will actually make you feel satisfied.

1½ cups whole wheat flour

2 tablespoons toasted wheat germ

2 teaspoons baking powder

½ teaspoon salt

2 eggs or ½ cup fat-free liquid egg substitute

1 cup low-fat plain yogurt

¼ cup firmly packed light brown sugar

2 tablespoons canola oil

1½ cups fresh or frozen (thawed) blueberries

Preheat the oven to 375°F, and coat a 12-cup muffin pan with cooking spray. In a large bowl, whisk together the flour, wheat germ, baking powder, and salt and set aside. Then, in a small bowl, whisk together the eggs or egg substitute and yogurt. Whisk in the sugar and oil.

Add to the flour mixture and stir just until the dry ingredients are moistened. Stir in the blueberries. Divide the batter among the muffin cups, filling each about two-thirds full.

Bake for 20 minutes, or until a wooden pick inserted in the center of a muffin comes out clean. Transfer to a rack and cool slightly. Store the muffins in a covered container for up to 1 day at room temperature or up to 1 month in the freezer.

**2-SECOND LIFE CHANGER**

Bananas help lend a thicker, creamier consistency to a smoothie. At the start of each week, dice a bunch of bananas and place them in a resealable plastic bag in your freezer. Not only will it save you prep time in the morning, but you won't have to add as much ice.

## GO GREEN

Kale, spinach, arugula, celery, fresh herbs like mint, parsley, and cilantro—there are few greens that you can't toss into your blender. (Okay, maybe broccoli. It's healthy and delicious in so many ways, but not as smoothie friendly.) If you find it hard to get your daily serving of greens, consider adding them to your smoothie. A handful of spinach might change the color, but it really won't alter the taste; however, sometimes veggies can be bitter, so shoot for a 70:30 fruit-to-greens ratio.

## FILL UP ON FIBER

Toss in hunger-squashing ingredients like wheat germ, ground flax-seed, and high-fiber fruits (think raspberries, blackberries, and avocado). Leave the peel on thin-skinned fruits such as pears and peaches.

## CONSISTENCY COUNTS

Ice adds thickness, but too much of it can dilute the flavor and water it down. Boost consistency with ingredients like avocado, low-fat Greek yogurt, frozen bananas, canned pumpkin, nonfat milk powder, and fruit. (Keep in mind that frozen fruits add more texture than fresh. Bonus: They're less expensive, too.)

## BE CREATIVE

There are no rules as to what's "allowed" in a smoothie. Experiment with different ingredients and spices to create surprisingly amazing combinations. (A personal favorite: frozen mixed berries, fresh grated ginger, spinach, baby carrots, and Greek yogurt.)

## WATCH FOR WANNABES

Forty-six percent of smoothie consumers also purchase these beverages away from home, usually from fast-food joints. You may feel good about your "healthy" choice, but most are filled with added sugar, high-calorie juices, and other processed ingredients.

# Lighten Up Your Lunches

▶ Whether you're eating lunch at home, the office, or on the go, this midday meal can either keep your metabolism humming or send you spiraling toward midafternoon cravings. Follow these simple tips and strategies to make smarter decisions during the day.

## Raise the (Salad) Bar

It's arguably the most utilized "diet" meal, but it presents two problems: Women either use the same, boring, super-light ingredients (so they don't feel satisfied by it), or they load up their lettuce with so many calorie-laden toppings that it hardly deserves to be categorized as a salad.

What's more, few foods differ more dramatically on the nutrition front than a heavy, overloaded chain restaurant salad and one made quickly but

 **2-SECOND LIFE CHANGER**

Make sure your lettuce is thoroughly washed, but also dried—a common step that most people overlook. Any water that remains on the leaves will prevent the dressing from adhering to the salad. A salad spinner works great, or just lay the leaves on paper towels.

carefully at home. Save your cash and conserve your precious calories—
and never leave your mouth underwhelmed or stomach growling—by
following these six simple rules to building a better salad.

## 1. GET CREATIVE WITH YOUR BASE

A salad doesn't have to start with iceberg (and probably shouldn't).
Robust dark greens add power nutrients such as folate and vitamins
A, C, and K for negligible calories, while the fiber and complex carbs in
whole grains fill you up.

Match your toppings to your lettuce. Sturdier leaves like iceberg and
romaine are fit to hold bulkier ingredients and thicker dressings, while
delicate lettuces like arugula and baby spinach tend to be best suited
for vinaigrettes and lighter toppings.

Try one of these:

- 1½ cups romaine, Bibb, frisée, spinach, or arugula (or any combination)
- ½ cup cooked grains, such as quinoa or whole grain couscous
- 1 to 2 ounces soba noodles or whole wheat linguine

## 2. PUMP UP THE PROTEIN

Protein provides the belly-filling satisfaction that transforms a side
salad into a main dish. Get your dose from lean sources such as
chicken, fish, beans, or tofu.

Try one of these:

- 2 ounces fish, such as smoked, canned, or fresh salmon; trout; or
  smoked bluefish
- 5 large shrimp (broiled, boiled, or grilled) or 2 ounces lump crabmeat
- 3 ounces skinless chicken breast, broiled or grilled
- ¼ to 1 cup cooked beans, such chickpeas, cannellini, or black beans
- 2 ounces marinated, cooked tofu

## 3. ADD COLOR

Vibrant produce doesn't just make your salad look pretty—it also ensures your dish is loaded with vitamins and other nutrients. Just one-quarter of a red bell pepper provides more than 40 percent of your daily vitamin A needs, while tomatoes are full of cancer-fighting lycopene.

Try one (or more!) of these:
- ¼ cup chopped red, yellow, or orange bell pepper
- ¼ to ½ cup chopped red, yellow, orange, or green tomato (about 1 medium)
- ¼ cup chopped red, golden, or Chioggia beet
- ¼ cup shredded carrot
- 1 or 2 medium slices red onion

## 4. TOSS IN SOMETHING SOFT

A touch of softness gives a salad balance and texture and makes it extra satisfying. A soft cheese also provides calcium and protein, plus a hint of saltiness. Just be mindful of how much you toss in: Cheese and other rich ingredients can ratchet up the calorie count.

Try one of these:
- 1 to 2 teaspoons soft cheese, such as feta, goat, or blue cheese
- ⅛ avocado
- 1 heart of palm

## 5. FIRE UP THE FLAVOR

Spicy, tart, or sweet ingredients add a layer of depth and complexity to a salad and can offset some of the more bitter greens and veggies. For example, fresh fruit will satisfy a sweet tooth, while zingy fresh herbs boost flavor but not fat.

Try one of these:
- ½ cup citrus fruit, such as fresh orange, lime, or grapefruit

- Tangy veggies, such as radishes, scallions, chives, grated or pickled ginger, or jalapeño chile pepper, to taste
- Zesty herbs, such as cilantro, basil, oregano, or tarragon, to taste

## 6. TOP IT OFF WITH SOME CRUNCH

Crispy, crunchy ingredients wake up your palate and are the perfect contrast to soft greens, noodles, and grains. Nuts and seeds are great choices because they can satisfy a raging appetite, and many, including sunflower and pumpkin seeds, are top sources of antioxidants and vitamins. Homemade croutons take minutes to make and contain a fraction of the fat and calories of store-bought varieties.

Try one of these:
- 1 to 2 teaspoons nuts, such as pecans, walnuts, peanuts, macadamia nuts, almonds, or pine nuts
- 1 to 2 teaspoons seeds, such as pumpkin, sunflower, sesame, or poppy
- ⅛ cup whole grain croutons (make your own by toasting a whole wheat baguette or pita)

KEEP IN MIND THE MOST IMPORTANT ELEMENT OF ANY SALAD: PORTIONS, PORTIONS, PORTIONS! YOU CAN NEVER HAVE TOO MUCH PRODUCE, BUT WATCH YOUR SERVING SIZES OF HIGH-CALORIE NUTS, CHEESES, AND DRESSINGS.

## *"The art of being wise is knowing what to overlook."*

—WILLIAM JAMES

# 9 SUPER SALADS

## Need some salad inspiration? Try one of these delicious and healthy combinations.

### APPLE-BLUE
Bibb lettuce
+
red onion
+
apple
+
blue cheese
+
grilled chicken
+
yogurt dressing

### THAI
buckwheat soba noodles
+
extra-firm tofu
+
carrots
+
red bell pepper
+
edamame
+
sesame seeds

### ASIAN
mixed greens
+
cucumber
+
mandarin oranges
+
chicken
+
almond slivers
+
ginger-soy dressing

### MEDITERRANEAN
arugula
+
tuna
+
hard-cooked egg
+
artichoke hearts
+
roasted peppers
+
olives
+
balsamic dressing

### CHOPPED
iceberg
+
hard-cooked egg
+
ham
+
cherry tomatoes
+
carrots
+
red onion
+
ranch dressing

### MOROCCAN
arugula
+
chickpeas
+
yellow tomato
+
cucumber
+
red onion
+
golden raisins
+
sunflower seeds

### BERRY CHICKEN
baby spinach
+
grilled chicken
+
strawberries
+
blueberries
+
yellow tomato
+
goat cheese crumbles
+
pecans

### SALMON
Bibb lettuce
+
canned salmon
+
avocado
+
pink grapefruit
+
red onion
+
beets
+
pistachios

### SHRIMP
romaine lettuce
+
shrimp
+
celery
+
red cabbage
+
grape tomatoes
+
blue cheese crumbles

# DIY with Mason Jar Dressings

Considering how easy it is to make vinaigrette at home, you don't have to settle for store-bought dressings that are loaded with salt and high-fructose corn syrup. Here are five delicious homemade dressings to try. You can use a bowl and whisk, but a clean mason jar is even better. Add your base flavorings and a vinegar and oil (no more than 2 parts oil to 1 part vinegar). Pour in the remaining seasonings and shake for 20 seconds. Store any leftovers in your fridge for up to a week.

*THAI*

1 tablespoon creamy peanut butter

2 tablespoons rice wine vinegar

2 tablespoons reduced-sodium soy sauce

2 tablespoons fresh lime juice

1 teaspoon firmly packed brown sugar

*CHILI SPICE*

1 tablespoon extra-virgin olive oil

2 tablespoons fresh orange juice

2 teaspoons white wine vinegar

½ teaspoon orange peel

½ teaspoon Dijon mustard

1 large pinch kosher salt

1 large pinch chili powder

 **SLIM-DOWN SECRET**

Toss out the fat-free vinaigrette: A study reported that fat enhances the absorption of compounds in veggies called carotenoids, which not only produce the vivid hues found in tomatoes, carrots, and bell peppers but also may reduce the risk for cancer, cardiovascular disease, and macular degeneration (vision loss). Researchers found that dressings containing monounsaturated fats maximized absorption (compared with saturated fats), which is good news if you're watching what you eat.

## 2-SECOND LIFE CHANGER

Don't throw out the last of your jam. Pour oil and vinegar directly into the jar, season with salt and pepper, and shake up semi-homemade berry vinaigrette in seconds.

### MOROCCAN

1 tablespoon olive oil

½ teaspoon orange peel

2 tablespoons lime juice

1 tablespoon honey

1 large pinch ground cinnamon

¼ teaspoon ground cumin

### BETTER BLUE CHEESE

1 teaspoon sugar

1½ teaspoons white wine vinegar

2 tablespoons water

2 tablespoons 0% plain Greek yogurt

2 tablespoons light canola
  mayonnaise

1 tablespoon blue cheese crumbles

### BERRY VINAIGRETTE

¼ cup sliced strawberries

1 tablespoon fresh orange juice

1½ teaspoons red wine vinegar

½ teaspoon orange peel

½ teaspoon sugar

2 tablespoons 0% plain Greek yogurt

1 large pinch kosher salt

 OUT TO LUNCH? ORDER A CHEF'S SALAD WITH OLIVE OIL AND BALSAMIC VINEGAR. THE LEAN PROTEIN, (TURKEY AND HAM) AND HEALTHY FATS (OLIVE OIL) HELP KEEP YOU BURNING FAT AND PREVENT A MIDDAY LULL. ORDER THE DRESSING ON THE SIDE TO REIN IN THE CALORIES.

# Slim Down with Soup

Bored with salad? Soup can be an equally fulfilling and slimming meal: According to a study published in the journal *Physiology & Behavior*, people consumed the fewest calories on days when they ate soup rather than the same ingredients in solid form. Another study published in *Appetite* found that people who started lunch with vegetable soup ended up eating 20 percent less than those who skipped the soup.

This cold-weather comfort food is an easy way to get your vegetables in, and it contains plenty of water to fill you up. Steer clear of those with the words *cream, bisque,* or *stew* in the name (they tend to be fattening). Instead, choose broth-based soups such as miso, chicken, or vegetable; noncream tomato-based soups; and bean or lentil soups. Use this cheat sheet to score a healthy option whether you're prepping from scratch, serving from a can, or grabbing to-go.

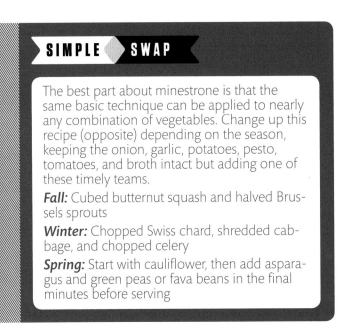

> **SIMPLE ▸ SWAP**
>
> The best part about minestrone is that the same basic technique can be applied to nearly any combination of vegetables. Change up this recipe (opposite) depending on the season, keeping the onion, garlic, potatoes, pesto, tomatoes, and broth intact but adding one of these timely teams.
>
> **Fall:** Cubed butternut squash and halved Brussels sprouts
>
> **Winter:** Chopped Swiss chard, shredded cabbage, and chopped celery
>
> **Spring:** Start with cauliflower, then add asparagus and green peas or fava beans in the final minutes before serving

# MINESTRONE WITH PESTO

Vary the specific vegetables depending on what's in your fridge and what looks good in the market, but be sure to finish with a spoonful of jarred pesto, which helps tie the whole bowl together.

1 tablespoon olive oil
1 medium onion, chopped
2 cloves garlic, minced
8 ounces Yukon gold or red potatoes, cubed
2 medium carrots, peeled and chopped
1 medium zucchini, chopped
8 ounces green beans, ends trimmed, halved
Salt
1 can (14 ounces) diced tomatoes
8 cups reduced-sodium chicken broth
½ teaspoon dried thyme
Black pepper
½ can (14–16 ounces) cannellini beans, drained
Pesto
Grated Parmesan cheese

*Heat the olive oil in a large pot over medium heat. Add the onion and garlic and cook until the onion is translucent, about 3 minutes. Stir in the potatoes, carrots, zucchini, and green beans. Season with a bit of salt and cook, stirring, for 3 to 4 minutes to release the vegetables' aromas. Add the tomatoes, broth, and thyme and turn the heat down to low.*

*Season with salt (if still needed) and pepper to taste. Simmer for at least 15 minutes, and up to 45. Before serving, stir in the beans and heat through. Serve with a dollop of pesto and a bit of grated Parmesan.*

MAKES 4 SERVINGS. PER SERVING: 200 CALORIES, 5 G TOTAL FAT, 1.5 G SATURATED FAT, 490 MG SODIUM

# BROCCOLI-CHEDDAR SOUP

This is definitely on my short list of favorite soups—even if, more often than not, it's remorsefully lacking in nutritional value. Most iterations of broccoli-cheese soup are made up of very little broccoli and a whole lot of cheese, which is why it's a great choice to make at home. This may take a little more prep work, but the calories you'll save by using flavorful, fresh ingredients in the right proportions (so tons of broccoli and only a handful of cheese) are worth the extra effort.

1 tablespoon butter
1 yellow onion, finely chopped
1 large carrot, finely chopped
1 head broccoli, cut into florets
2 cloves garlic, chopped
1 tablespoon flour
1 cup reduced-sodium chicken broth
1 cup beer
2 cups low-fat milk
1 cup (4 ounces) shredded sharp Cheddar cheese
Salt and black pepper
Tabasco sauce
4 Parmesan cheese crisps

*Heat the butter in a large pot over medium heat. Add the onion, carrot, broccoli, and garlic and cook for 5 minutes, or until the vegetables soften. Stir in the flour and cook until it evenly coats all of the vegetables. Add the broth and beer, stirring vigorously to keep the flour from clumping. Simmer for a few minutes, then pour the mixture (working in batches, if need be) into a blender and puree until mostly smooth (a bit of texture can be nice here). You can also use a hand blender to puree the soup in the pot.*

*Return the soup to the pot and bring to a simmer over low heat. Stir in the milk and cheese. After the cheese has fully melted into the soup, season with salt and pepper and a few good shakes of Tabasco. Serve each bowl of soup with a Parmesan crisp floating in the middle.*

MAKES 4 SERVINGS. PER SERVING: 290 CALORIES, 17 G TOTAL FAT, 9 G SATURATED FAT, 580 MG SODIUM

## AMY'S ORGANIC BLACK BEAN CHILI

Half a can of chili might seem like a small lunch, but if you're worried it won't fill your stomach, don't be. Each serving is packed with fiber and protein.

PER SERVING (½ CAN): 200 CALORIES, 13 G PROTEIN, 31 G CARBOHYDRATES, 3 G TOTAL FAT, 0 G SATURATED FAT, 13 G FIBER, 680 MG SODIUM

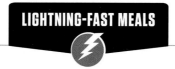

### LIGHTNING-FAST MEALS

Add a sprinkle of cheese, a few thin slices of avocado, and a few scoops of plain Greek yogurt to make this chili a complete meal.

## CAMPBELL'S SELECT HARVEST HEALTHY REQUEST MEXICAN-STYLE CHICKEN TORTILLA SOUP

This is as light as soup gets. You can slurp the whole veggie-loaded can for 100 calories and not worry about serving-size overload.

PER CUP: 50 CALORIES, 3 G PROTEIN, 0 G TOTAL FAT, 0 G SATURATED FAT, 4 G FIBER, 480 MG SODIUM

## AU BON PAIN'S TOMATO RICE SOUP

The calories are commendably low and it carries one of the lowest sodium counts you'll likely ever encounter in a commercially prepared soup.

PER SERVING (LARGE): 170 CALORIES, 2 G TOTAL FAT, 0 G SATURATED FAT, 390 MG SODIUM

## WENDY'S CHILI

Slightly higher in sodium, yes, but with lots of protein and minimal calories, this may be the best drive-thru soup out there.

PER SERVING (SMALL): 210 CALORIES, 17 G PROTEIN, 6 G TOTAL FAT, 2.5 G SATURATED FAT, 880 MG SODIUM

# Build a Better Sandwich

If salads are the go-to pick for weight-conscious women, sandwiches may be the antithesis. But it's not the two slices of bread that are ruining this lunchtime staple—it's everything in between them. Deli sandwiches, for example, often have enough meat for two lunches and are loaded with extra fat, sodium, and calories. Save your money (and your waistline) by making your own using these five rules.

## STACK UP

Sandwich architecture is essential. Wet ingredients like tomatoes and roasted peppers go in the center of the sandwich to prevent the bread from getting soggy. Lettuce and cheese go against the bread for protection.

## WATCH THE HEAT WAVE

Even if you want that toasted taste and texture, toasting your bread can sometimes make a sandwich too tough to eat. Instead, sear each slice on one side in a skillet over medium-high heat until browned and crisp. (You can also toast one side under the broiler for a few minutes.) Stack the sandwich with the toasted sides facing in—it won't scratch the roof of your mouth and the toasty barrier will prevent sogginess.

## DECODE THE DELI

Not all meats are created equal. Sliced whole-roasted ham, turkey, and pot roast are known in deli-speak as "whole cuts." Far more common, though, are processed meats, which tend to be fattier and are made by adding preservatives (mostly salt) and sometimes fillers to ground meat. You can usually recognize processed meats by their unnaturally uniform shape (think bologna, salami, capicola)—the better to fit on a bun. The best way to make sure you're getting a whole cut is to ask for it.

**GOOD:** HONEY HAM. CONTAINS TWO-THIRDS THE PROTEIN OF ROAST BEEF, BUT IS STILL FAIRLY LOW IN FAT AND CALORIES. IT HAS ABOUT 15 MORE CALORIES PER SERVING, SO PAIR WITH LOW-CALORIE CONDIMENTS.

**BETTER:** ROAST BEEF. LEAN AND LOW IN SODIUM, DELIVERING 7 GRAMS OF PROTEIN PER SLICE.

**BEST:** TURKEY. PILE IT HIGH. EACH SLICE HAS 6 GRAMS OF PROTEIN AND ONLY 30 CALORIES.

## CHOOSE YOUR CHEESE WISELY

Ask for your order to be thinly sliced—not only will you save calories, but thin cheese slices are a better choice for hot sandwiches. And don't overdo it: Three slices of meat or one slice of cheese is 1 serving.

**GOOD:** SHARP CHEDDAR. CONTAINS ABOUT THE SAME AMOUNT OF CALORIES AS SWISS, BUT IS HIGHER IN SODIUM.

**BETTER:** SWISS. HAS 83 PERCENT LESS SODIUM THAN AMERICAN, AND ABOUT 25 PERCENT OF THE RECOMMENDED DAILY VALUE OF CALCIUM.

**BEST:** FRESH MOZZARELLA. HAS A GREAT BALANCE OF PROTEIN AND FAT, AND ENOUGH SUBSTANCE TO ACT AS A STAND-IN FOR MEAT.

## GET CREATIVE WITH CONDIMENTS

Too many great spreads go overlooked while mayo and oil and vinegar drive calorie counts through the roof. Try pesto, hummus, or even cranberry spread on your next sandwich. Just remember to watch the portions—1 to 2 tablespoons is the sweet spot.

**GOOD:** GUACAMOLE. SWAP AVOCADO FOR MAYO FOR A HEALTHIER FAT CONTENT. GUACAMOLE IS GREAT WITH TURKEY AND SWISS.

**BETTER:** HONEY MUSTARD. IS LOW IN CALORIES AND PACKED WITH FLAVOR. SLATHER IT ON TOASTED WHEAT BREAD, AND ADD HAM, SLICED APPLE, AND BRIE CHEESE.

**BEST:** HUMMUS. PACKS A LOAD OF FIBER AND A MAYO-LIKE RICHNESS WITHOUT THE CALORIES. TRY COMBINING IT WITH ROAST BEEF AND ROASTED RED PEPPERS.

# 4 SUPER SANDWICHES

Save some cash (and precious calories) by stacking one of these tasty sandwiches at home.

| POWER-UP PITA | BLTE | VEGAPALOOZA | MEXI-MELT |
|---|---|---|---|
| whole grain pita | toasted sourdough | ciabatta | English muffin |
| + | + | + | + |
| hummus | arugula | grilled vegetables | grilled chicken or turkey |
| + | + | + | + |
| roast beef | tomato | roasted peppers | Jack cheese |
| + | + | + | + |
| romaine | bacon | pesto | avocado |
| + | + | + | + |
| onion | sunny-side-up egg | fresh mozzarella | salsa |
| + | | | |
| tomato | | | |

# Salad Sandwich Makeover

Chicken, egg, tuna—they're inexpensive staples, but for all the protein-loaded, metabolism-boosting potential, when combined into a "salad," they are not often thought of as a weight-loss ally (thanks to the massive amount of mayo). Recreate the old standbys for a healthier, more delicious variation. Make a big batch on Sunday and divvy it up for lunches and snacks throughout the week. Greek yogurt binds every bit as well as mayo, for about one-eighth the calories. It's so rich you may not even notice a difference.

## THREE RULES FOR A SKINNIER DELI SALAD

1. **Don't drown it.** You want just enough binder to lightly coat your ingredients. If you can't distinguish the individual ingredients in the salad, you've gone way too far.
2. **Think about texture.** Like a regular salad, protein-based salads benefit from crunch. Toasted nuts, celery, and apples are all excellent choices.
3. **Partner up.** Switch up what you pair the salad with. Have it over a bed of lettuce, on an open-faced English muffin, or with carrots or wheat crackers.

## FOUR FRESH DELI SALAD COMBOS

| CURRIED CHICKEN | RIVIERA SALMON | TUSCAN TUNA | FIERY EGG SALAD |
|---|---|---|---|
| Chicken | Salmon | Tuna | Hard-cooked eggs |
| + onion | + olive oil | + celery | + onion |
| + carrot | + Dijon mustard | + olives | + pickle |
| + golden raisins | + capers | + sun-dried tomatoes | +mayo |
| + mayo | + fresh parsley or dill | + olive oil | + Sriracha or hot sauce |
| + curry powder | | + lemon juice | |

# At Dinner . . .

➤ There's a saying that goes something like "eat breakfast like a king, lunch like a prince, and dinner like a pauper." The instinctive translation: Breakfast is the most important meal of the day. (I think it's more to speak to portion size than meal quality.) Here's the problem with all the attention on your a.m. eating: A survey found that the healthiness of the food we eat decreases 1.7 percent for every hour that passes in the day. Other research reports that dinner is 15.9 percent less healthy than breakfast on average.

The good news: This section is packed full of fat-fighting, hunger-squashing meal ideas that are super simple to prepare and will whittle your waistline without stripping your wallet.

## Skewer Your Way Slim

The very idea of a kebab—lean meat or fish skewered with fresh vegetables and lightly brushed with sauce or dusted with spices—makes it one of your most trusted waist-trimming allies (and should make it one of your dinner staples). Plus, they take just a few minutes to assemble and can be prepared ahead of time. (Not to mention, any leftovers can be used to make a great salad or sandwich.) Use these simple steps to build a better kebab.

### STEP 1

Soak wooden skewers in water for at least 20 minutes before loading them up. The moisture will prevent the wood from catching fire and scorching your dinner.

### STEP 2

The protein you're cooking will determine the size of the produce on your skewers. Shrimp and scallops cook quickly, so fruits and veggies

# SKEWER YOUR WAY SLIM

Try one of these perfectly crafted kebabs, or use the list below of the healthiest mix-and-match ingredients for the perfect calorie-crushing combo.

| **TERIYAKI SALMON** | **PESTO CHICKEN** | **MEDITERRANEAN SCALLOP** | **JERK PORK** |
|:---:|:---:|:---:|:---:|
| salmon | chicken | scallops | pork |
| + | + | + | + |
| mushrooms | cherry tomatoes | zucchini | onions |
| + | + | + | + |
| pineapple | zucchini | onions | red bell peppers |
| + | + | + | + |
| onions | pesto | tapenade | peaches |
| + | | | + |
| teriyaki | | | jerk sauce |

### PROTEIN

- ✓ Chicken breast or thigh
- ✓ Lean beef (sirloin or tenderloin is best)
- ✓ Pork loin
- ✓ Pork tenderloin
- ✓ Salmon
- ✓ Shrimp (peeled, deveined)

### PRODUCE

- ✓ Cherry tomatoes
- ✓ Chopped bell peppers
- ✓ Chopped onions
- ✓ Chopped zucchini
- ✓ Cubed pineapple and peaches
- ✓ Mushrooms
- ✓ Sliced eggplant

### SAUCE

- ✓ Barbecue sauce
- ✓ Jerk sauce
- ✓ Olive oil, lemon, and herbs
- ✓ Olive tapenade
- ✓ Pesto
- ✓ Teriyaki

should be cut smaller. Chicken and pork take time, so pair them with larger chunks.

## STEP 3

You can marinate the loaded skewers in sauce before grilling—up to 2 hours for meat, but no more than 30 minutes for seafood. Or simply brush the sauce onto the food before grilling and at least once during cooking. Whether the food has been marinated or not, it's always great to finish the kebabs with a light brush of fresh sauce just before bringing them to the table.

## STEP 4

You want a medium-hot grill—not so hot that it chars the food's outside before cooking the inside, but hot enough that the food's surface will fully caramelize.

# "Believe you can and you're halfway there."

—THEODORE ROOSEVELT

# Flip a Better Burger

I was a horribly picky (and, my parents would probably say, illogical) eater growing up. I ate meat, but beef never made the cut. This meant my entrée options at summer cookouts were limited to hot dogs—or sometimes a frozen veggie burger that someone happened to have in the freezer.

I have since graduated to accepting ground beef in things like chili and tacos, but patties are still a no-fly zone. I know I'm missing out: With minimal effort (and ingredients), you can whip up a protein-packed dinner in just minutes. Thankfully, the burger platform is so incredibly versatile, and chefs and restaurants everywhere are playing with different ingredients and flavors in their patties—including different meat (and meatless) variations. Shake up your standard burger with these mouthwatering, super-simple alternatives that will help you shed pounds while keeping you totally satisfied.

## SALMON BURGER

12-ounce salmon fillet
1 teaspoon finely chopped fresh rosemary
⅓ cup panko bread crumbs
1 egg white
2 teaspoons lemon peel

*Preheat the grill. Cut the salmon into pieces and pulse in a food processor for 1 minute. Combine in a medium bowl with the remaining ingredients and form into 4 patties. Grill for 4 to 5 minutes, then flip and grill for another 4 to 5 minutes.*

MAKES 4 SERVINGS. PER SERVING: 165 CALORIES, 21 G PROTEIN, 6 G CARBOHYDRATES, 6 G TOTAL FAT, 1 G SATURATED FAT, 1 G FIBER, 295 MG SODIUM

## TURKEY BURGER

12 ounces ground turkey
2 tablespoons Dijon mustard
2 tablespoons finely minced shallot
2 tablespoons chopped fresh parsley

*Preheat the grill. Combine all the ingredients in a medium bowl and form into 4 patties. Grill for 5 to 6 minutes, then flip and grill for another 5 to 6 minutes, or until the burgers reach an internal temperature of 165°F and the meat is no longer pink.*

MAKES 4 SERVINGS. PER SERVING: 170 CALORIES, 17 G PROTEIN, 8 G CARBOHYDRATES, 9 G TOTAL FAT, 2 G SATURATED FAT, 1 G FIBER, 240 MG SODIUM

# BLACK BEAN BURGER

1½ cups canned no-salt-added black beans, rinsed and drained
½ yellow bell pepper, sliced
⅓ cup course chopped red onion
¾ cup shredded carrot
⅓ cup dry quick-cooking oats
2½ teaspoons canola oil
½ teaspoon ground cumin

*Preheat the grill. Put all the ingredients in a food processor and pulse until combined, 2 to 3 minutes. Form into 4 patties. Mist a piece of foil with cooking spray and place the foil on the grill. Cook the patties on the foil for 5 minutes, then flip and cook for 5 minutes more.*

MAKES 4 SERVINGS. PER SERVING: 170 CALORIES, 7 G PROTEIN, 25 G CARBOHYDRATES, 6 G TOTAL FAT, 0 G SATURATED FAT, 6 G FIBER, 70 MG SODIUM

# BISON BURGER

This sweet-tasting meat gives you all the satisfaction of a traditional burger, but with only 7 grams of fat and about 150 calories per serving.

12 ounces ground grass-fed bison
½ cup chopped onion
½ teaspoon garlic powder
¼ teaspoon smoked paprika

*Preheat the grill. Combine all the ingredients in a medium bowl and form into 4 patties. Grill for 5 to 6 minutes, then flip and grill for another 5 to 6 minutes, or until the burgers reach an internal temperature of 155°F.*

MAKES 4 SERVINGS. PER SERVING: 145 CALORIES, 18 G PROTEIN, 3 G CARBOHYDRATES, 7 G TOTAL FAT, 2.5 G SATURATED FAT, 1 G FIBER, 90 MG SODIUM

# 4 Rules for a Perfect Patty

Most are quick to blame the grilling technique when a burger is dry and dense, but the real culprit is often how the patty was made in the first place. Whether you're using beef, turkey, or tuna, these four steps will make it better.

## RULE 1

Mix the meat and other ingredients lightly by hand until just blended—then stop. Overhandling can cause meat to turn tough. When working with legumes, puree only half and then lightly mix in the rest. This will help the burgers hold together on the grill.

## RULE 2

Lean meats like chicken need extra moisture from the inside, so mold the patties around cheese or salsa. Or build your burgers around an ice cube to keep them moist.

## RULE 3

When forming the burger patties, make them uniform in both size and thickness so they'll cook in the same amount of time. Press your thumb into the center of a meat patty to form a quarter-inch depression. The meat will expand during cooking to fill the indentation, which will keep the burger flat and help it cook evenly.

## RULE 4

Lightly coat patties with olive or vegetable oil to lock in the juices and prevent sticking.

# TOP IT OFF

Go beyond ketchup and mustard—these ingredients boost the flavor of America's most popular protein patty.

- ✓ Asian chili paste
- ✓ Chopped caramelized shallots
- ✓ Chopped chipotle peppers
- ✓ Chopped green olives
- ✓ Chopped sun-dried tomatoes
- ✓ Creole seasoning
- ✓ Finely chopped toasted pecans
- ✓ Pesto

# Get Hooked

Low in calories, packed with protein, and a leading source of powerful omega-3s—seafood should top every grocery list. Yet women still don't get the recommended two servings a week. Why? Either they don't know how to cook seafood or they're concerned about things like mercury or chemical pollutants. Start small with these two options that are low in mercury, packed with nutrients, and a cinch to prepare.

 **SLIM DOWN SECRET**

Salmon's omega-3s slow digestion and delay hunger, and one study found that they may also target belly fat: Women who ate a balanced diet that included omega-3s lost 1.5 pounds more of torso fat than women on the same diet without the omega-3s.

## SALMON

This mild, pink-fleshed fish is well known for its hefty omega-3 content, which gives a rich flavor; it's also a great source of vitamin D, which is essential for strong bones and a healthy immune system. Just 3 ounces contain 52 percent of your recommended daily dose of niacin, a B vitamin that boosts energy and helps your body metabolize carbs and fat. You'll get the most flavor from wild-caught species, such as Alaskan king.

**BEST WITH:** light flavors such as citrus or soy to balance its substantial flavor. It pairs nicely with slightly acidic greens like bok choy or spinach, which offset its richness.

# ORANGE-MAPLE SALMON

*Whisk together ¼ cup orange juice, 1 tablespoon maple syrup, 1 tablespoon soy sauce, and ½ teaspoon minced garlic. Pour over a 4-ounce salmon fillet and marinate for 15 minutes. Grill for 8 to 10 minutes, flipping halfway through.*

PER FILLET: 253 CALORIES, 24 G PROTEIN, 21 G CARBOHYDRATES, 7 G TOTAL FAT, 1 G SATURATED FAT, 0 G FIBER, 443 MG SODIUM

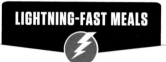

## LIGHTNING-FAST MEALS

### THREE SIMPLE TWEAKS, THREE SIMPLE SALMON DISHES:

| **1** | **2** | **3** |
|---|---|---|
| 2 tablespoons hoisin sauce, 2 tablespoons reduced-sodium soy sauce, 2 tablespoons orange juice | 2 tablespoons Dijon mustard, 2 tablespoons honey, ½ tablespoon chili powder | 2 tablespoons softened butter, 1 tablespoon canned chipotle pepper, lime juice |

## SCALLOPS

These petite mollusks are one of the leanest proteins around, with only 95 calories and less than 1 gram of fat per 3 ounces. They also contain 20 percent of the immune-boosting selenium you need in a day. Bay scallops are soft, sweet, and more delicate tasting compared to steaklike sea scallops. (Both are equally delicious and take just minutes to prepare.)

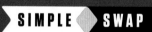

### SIMPLE SWAP

Sea scallops in the seafood case can be pricey, but scallops rarely arrive at the market fresh. Instead, they're frozen after catching and defrosted when put on sale. So why pay extra for them when you can buy them frozen for less? Grocers like Trader Joe's and Whole Foods sell bags of high-quality scallops and shrimp for about 60 percent of the typical cost. Avoid scallops treated in sodium tripolyphosphate, a soaking solution that causes scallops to absorb a lot of liquid so they weigh—and cost—more.

**BEST WITH:** subtle Mediterranean flavors, such as white wine, zesty lemon, capers, rosemary, or tomatoes. Add to a fiery pasta dish to pump up the meal.

## SCALLOPS FRA DIAVOLO

*Heat 1 teaspoon olive oil in a medium saucepan over medium heat. Add ½ clove minced garlic and 3 ounces bay scallops. Sauté for 1 minute. Add ½ cup canned fire-roasted tomatoes and a pinch of red-pepper flakes. Sauté for 1 minute more. Toss with 1 cup cooked whole wheat spaghetti and top with 1 tablespoon chopped fresh basil.*

PER RECIPE: 322 CALORIES, 23 G PROTEIN, 46 G CARBOHYDRATES, 6 G TOTAL FAT, 1 G SATURATED FAT, 7 G FIBER, 432 MG SODIUM

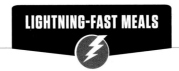

### LIGHTNING-FAST MEALS

In a skillet over medium heat, cook frozen veggies with 1 to 2 tablespoons soy sauce, 1 teaspoon olive oil, and a pinch of firmly packed brown sugar for 10 minutes. Add frozen cooked shrimp (slightly thawed) and cook for 5 more minutes.

# Something Smells Fishy!

The downside to cooking seafood: One meal can make your kitchen stink for days. Minimize unwelcome odors with these five tips.

### 1. GO FISH

Tilapia, snapper, and halibut tend to have less of a smell. And, of course, the fresher the fish, the less odor it has, so be sure to ask what just came in that day.

### 2. MILK IT

Soaking fillets in milk for a half hour before cooking can help cut down on the smell.

### 3. TURN DOWN THE HEAT

Low-heat cooking methods release the fewest odors, so instead of frying or broiling, try poaching, baking, or steaming (the lid will help hold in the fishy aroma).

### 4. JUICE UP

Most fish is served with lemon for a good reason: Not only does the citrus add flavor (for almost no calories), but its acidic juices also act as a natural deodorizer. Squeeze some on your fillet, and after cooking rub extra lemon wedges on your hands, knives, and cutting boards to cut the fishy stench. Dressing fish with cumin or curry is another great way to mask the odor, because these spices have their own powerful aromas.

### 5. CLEAN UP IMMEDIATELY

Wash the dishes and bag up any scraps. Then, simmer a pot of water with vinegar (or cinnamon, if you prefer) on the stove for about 20 minutes to squelch any stench.

# Fish in a Flash

Forgot to defrost a fillet before heading off to work? Use these three steps to take fish from freezer to plate in 15 minutes.

1. Preheat the oven to 450°F. Rinse the frozen fillet under cold water to remove any ice, then pat it dry. Brush both sides of the fillet with olive oil, place on a foil-lined baking sheet, and put the sheet on the top rack of the oven.
2. Sprinkle any combination of spices onto the fish 4 minutes into cooking. (If you do this earlier, the spices won't stick to the frozen flesh.)
3. Cook the seasoned fillet for another 8 to 11 minutes. Once the fish is opaque throughout, remove it from the oven and enjoy!

# Fight Fat with Flavor!

Healthy cooking doesn't have to be bland and boring. Use these cooking solutions to ramp up a meal without sending the calorie count soaring.

## SKINNY SAUCES

## BALSAMIC REDUCTION

GREAT ON: Pork, chicken breasts, or swordfish steaks as a sticky, flavorful glaze, and just about all vegetables, which will benefit from the sweet-and-sour combo of sugar and vinegar. Blend this balsamic reduction with some herbs and a few teaspoons of olive oil and it doubles as a marinade.

1 tablespoon canola oil
1 small red onion, thinly sliced
3 tablespoons firmly packed
    dark brown sugar
½ teaspoon salt
½ teaspoon black pepper
2 cups balsamic vinegar

*Heat the oil in a medium skillet or saucepan over medium-high heat until shimmering. Add the onion, sugar, salt, and pepper and cook, stirring until softened, about 3 minutes. Add the vinegar and bring to a boil.*

*Reduce the heat to medium and simmer, stirring often, for 30 minutes or until the vinegar has a syrupy consistency and has reduced to 1 cup.*

MAKES 8 SERVINGS (1 CUP TOTAL). PER SERVING: 100 CALORIES, 0 G PROTEIN, 17 G CARBOHYDRATES, 2 G TOTAL FAT, 0 G SATURATED FAT, 0 G FIBER, 160 MG SODIUM

## PEANUT SATAY

GREAT ON: Chicken, tofu, or pork skewers or any Asian-style noodle or rice dish. It's also a tasty dipping sauce for spring rolls. Swap smooth peanut butter for chunky to give your sauce some added substance. You can use other nut butters for variety, too.

¾ cup creamy peanut butter
½ cup light coconut milk
3 tablespoons reduced-sodium soy sauce
2 tablespoons freshly grated ginger
2 tablespoons mirin or rice wine
1 tablespoon lime juice
2 teaspoons hot sauce, such as Sriracha,
    or more to taste

*Whisk all the ingredients together in a bowl until smooth. Serve.*

MAKES 8 SERVINGS (1⅓ CUPS TOTAL). PER SERVING: 120 CALORIES, 5 G PROTEIN, 6 G CARBOHYDRATES, 9 G TOTAL FAT, 2.5 G SATURATED FAT, 1 G FIBER, 340 MG SODIUM

# ARUGULA CHIMICHURRI

GREAT ON: Grilled steak and grilled tuna steaks. If you want to get creative, add some to a potato dish—the herbs brighten up starchy spuds.

2 cups packed arugula (2½ ounces)
1 cup flat-leaf parsley (1 ounce)
1 teaspoon red-pepper flakes
½ cup extra-virgin olive oil
⅓ cup red wine vinegar
3 cloves garlic, minced
½ teaspoon salt
½ teaspoon freshly ground black pepper

*In a food processor, pulse the arugula and parsley until finely chopped. Transfer the chopped herbs to a bowl and whisk in the red-pepper flakes, olive oil, red wine vinegar, garlic, salt, and pepper.*

*Cover with plastic wrap and let stand at room temperature for 1 hour to allow the flavors to meld before serving.*

MAKES 12 SERVINGS (1 CUP TOTAL). PER SERVING: 90 CALORIES, 0 G PROTEIN, 1 G CARBOHYDRATES, 9 G TOTAL FAT, 1.5 G SATURATED FAT, 0 G FIBER, 100 MG SODIUM

# SMOOTH MOVES

Cooking is as much about your ability to adapt and improvise as it is about the recipe. Here are four genius fixes for some common snafus.

### IF IT'S . . . Runny
Cook it longer. Heat helps sauces thicken, and temperatures can vary, so keep cooking the sauce until it acquires a syruplike thickness.

### IF IT'S . . . Still Runny
You can add more cornstarch or flour if the recipe uses it, but to avoid lumps, first combine the cornstarch with warm water or broth. Add slowly to get your desired consistency.

### IF IT'S . . . Lumpy
Add liquids in a slow, steady stream while whisking vigorously. Make sure liquids are warm before pouring them in. If lumps remain, strain them out using a fine-mesh sieve.

### IF IT'S . . . Thick
Add more of whatever liquid is called for in the recipe, a small amount at a time, stirring until it is incorporated.

# ROMESCO SAUCE

GREAT ON: Grilled white-fleshed fish and shellfish, and raw or roasted vegetables—especially spring onions—whose milder flavor won't compete with this chunky Spanish condiment's nutty, full-bodied taste.

1 dried ancho chile pepper, soaked in
   boiling water for 30 minutes, seeds
   and stem removed
1 cup jarred roasted red peppers
¾ cup canned plum tomatoes,
   drained and crushed
5 cloves garlic, smashed
1 slice hearty white bread, torn into pieces
1 teaspoon smoked paprika
¼ cup olive oil
Salt and pepper to taste
⅓ cup toasted slivered almonds
2 tablespoons sherry vinegar

*Preheat the oven to 450°F. Toss the chile pepper, red peppers, tomatoes, garlic, bread, and paprika together on a foil-lined baking sheet. Drizzle with the oil and season with the salt and pepper. Roast until the peppers are slightly charred, 10 to 12 minutes.*

*Allow to cool, then place the mixture in a food processor. Add the almonds and vinegar and pulse until pureed. If the sauce is too thick, add water until it is the consistency of dip, thick but spreadable.*

MAKES 10 SERVINGS (1⅓ CUPS TOTAL). PER SERVING:
100 CALORIES, 2 G PROTEIN, 7 G CARBOHYDRATES,
7 G TOTAL FAT, 1 G SATURATED FAT, 1 G FIBER,
320 MG SODIUM

# SWEET WHOLE GRAIN MUSTARD SAUCE

GREAT ON: Salmon, shrimp, oven-fried panko-crusted chicken tenderloins, ham, and asparagus, all of which can stand up to this sauce's intense tanginess. Puree this sauce in a blender and you've got a perfect homemade sandwich spread.

1 tablespoon canola oil
½ cup minced shallots
6 tablespoons honey
¾ cup whole grain mustard
2 tablespoons cider vinegar
¼ teaspoon white pepper
Salt to taste

*Heat the oil in a skillet over medium-high heat. Add the shallots and cook, stirring, until softened, about 3 minutes. Add the honey and remove from heat. Stir in the mustard, vinegar, and white pepper; season with the salt.*

MAKES 6 SERVINGS (1½ CUPS TOTAL). PER SERVING:
74 CALORIES, 0 G PROTEIN, 14 G CARBOHYDRATES,
3 G TOTAL FAT, 0 G SATURATED FAT, 0 G FIBER,
390 MG SODIUM

## SPICE RUBS

If you're short on time, marinating your meat for 30 minutes or longer won't cut it. Instead, use a dry rub, which can sear flavors right into the meat in just a few minutes. Not only is this quicker, but it also kicks up the flavor without adding a lot of fat to your meal. The best part is, there's no hard-and-fast rule on the perfect rub. Just mix the spices together, pat all over beef or chicken, then cook as instructed. Tweak and refine your own blends based on your personal preferences and what you have in the pantry. Or use this cheat sheet to get you

# SEASON MORE, EAT LESS

Turns out, strong food aromas can help you eat 5 to 10 percent less of a meal, according to research published in the journal *Flavour*. Study authors explain that people may unconsciously take smaller bites to regulate the amount of flavor they experience. Try one of these scent-enhancing combos.

**ROSEMARY SALMON.** Combine 2 teaspoons olive oil and ½ teaspoon chopped fresh rosemary. Brush onto a salmon fillet and broil.

**HERB AND SPICE CHILI.** Stir ¼ teaspoon Chinese five-spice powder into 1 cup prepared chili. Add 1 teaspoon finely chopped fresh cilantro.

**GINGER-APPLE OATMEAL.** Cook ½ cup oats in 1 cup simmering fresh apple juice with 1 teaspoon freshly grated ginger.

**MINT CHICKEN.** Marinate a chicken breast in 1 tablespoon each of olive oil, plain Greek yogurt, and chopped fresh mint, then cook.

started—simply incorporate a seasoning from at least three of these groups into your mix.

**SALT** kosher salt, garlic salt, onion salt
**HEAT** black pepper, ground red pepper, chili powder, mustard powder
**SWEET** sugar, brown sugar, ground cinnamon
**SMOKE** ground cumin, smoked paprika
**HERBAL** oregano, thyme, rosemary, basil, dill

*THREE PERFECT BLENDS*
**FOR BEEF:** salt and pepper, garlic salt, ground red pepper, ground cumin, pinch of ground cinnamon
**FOR CHICKEN:** salt and pepper, ground cumin, chili powder, brown sugar
**FOR FISH:** salt and pepper, smoked paprika, thyme

 **2-SECOND LIFE CHANGER**

Is the meat done yet? The answer's in the palm of your hands. Hold your hand in front of you, palm up. Keeping your hand relaxed, touch your thumb and index finger together. Now, press the fleshy area under your thumb with a finger from your other hand. That's what rare feels like. Now, press your thumb and middle finger together—the fleshy area under your thumb now feels like medium cooked meat. Repeat with your ring finger for medium-well, and your pinky for well done. Now that you know what it should feel like, press the top of the meat (quickly!) with your finger as it's cooking. This trick works for boneless chicken (always cook well done) and red-meat steaks and chops (like pork and lamb).

# HERB-ROASTED TURKEY BREAST

8 cups water
¾ cup salt
1 cup sugar
1 large boneless turkey breast (3 pounds)
2 cloves garlic, peeled
Salt to taste
1 tablespoon olive oil
½ tablespoon finely chopped fresh rosemary
Black pepper to taste

*Combine the water, salt, and sugar in a pot large enough to hold the turkey and bring to a boil. Stir until the sugar and salt have fully dissolved. Remove from the heat and let cool to room temperature. Add the turkey breast, cover, and place in the fridge to brine for at least 4 hours, and up to overnight.*

*Preheat the oven to 425°F. Remove the turkey from the brine, pat dry, and roll up into a tight log. Use butcher twine to tie three separate knots, about 2" apart, that will hold the turkey in this tight shape.*

*Finely mince the garlic, using a pinch of salt and the back of your knife to mash it into a paste. Combine with the olive oil and rosemary, then rub all over the turkey, along with a good amount of black pepper. Place the turkey in a large roasting pan and roast for 1 hour, or until a thermometer inserted into the center reads 170°F and the juices run clear. Let the turkey rest before slicing.*

MAKES 12 SERVINGS. PER SERVING: 140 CALORIES, 2 G TOTAL FAT, 0 G SATURATED FAT, 520 MG SODIUM

## LEFTOVER LOVE

THERE'S A BIT OF PREP WORK INVOLVED, BUT ROASTED TURKEY WAS BUILT FOR LEFTOVERS, SO PLAN AHEAD: PREP THE TURKEY ON SATURDAY AND COOK IT SUNDAY. SERVE IT UP FOR SUNDAY DINNER WITH TRADITIONAL SIDES, THEN SAVE THE REST IN THE FRIDGE FOR UP TO A WEEK FOR NO-FUSS MEALS:

As a sandwich, stacked on sourdough with avocado, romaine, and whipped cream cheese cut with cranberry sauce

As a salad, tossed with arugula or spinach and hard-cooked egg slices, olives, and cherry tomatoes

As a taco, tossed with a few big spoonfuls of salsa verde, tucked into a warm tortilla, and topped with guacamole

# SIRLOIN STEAKS WITH SHALLOT-MUSTARD SAUCE

4 boneless sirloin steaks (4 or 5 ounces each)
1 teaspoon salt
½ teaspoon freshly ground black pepper
4 teaspoons extra-virgin olive oil
1 tablespoon Dijon mustard
2 tablespoons fresh lemon juice
1 large shallot, finely chopped

*Preheat the grill or broiler. Season the steaks on both sides with the salt and pepper, and brush with 1 teaspoon of the oil. Grill or broil for 3 to 4 minutes per side or until a thermometer inserted in the center registers 145°F for medium-rare. Meanwhile, in a small bowl, whisk together the mustard, lemon juice, shallot, and the remaining 3 teaspoons of oil. Place the steaks on plates and drizzle evenly with the sauce.*

MAKES 4 SERVINGS. PER SERVING: 207 CALORIES, 25 G PROTEIN, 3 G CARBOHYDRATES, 10 G TOTAL FAT, 3 G SATURATED FAT, 0 G FIBER, 446 MG SODIUM

LEFTOVER LOVE

MAKE A STEAK SANDWICH OR SALAD, USING THE SHALLOT-MUSTARD SAUCE AS YOUR SPREAD OR DRESSING.

# 50 Ways to Cook Better Chicken

At 110 calories and an impressive 23 grams of protein, skinless, boneless chicken breast clocks in as one of the most revered fat-burning foods you can eat. But without the right prep work, chicken can be, well, pretty boring. Take your pick of 50 mouthwatering recipes that taste too good to be good for your waistline.

## STIR-FRY

For a stir-fry, cut a raw chicken breast into bite-size pieces or thin strips. Cook the chicken in a nonstick skillet over medium-high heat until browned (3 to 5 minutes), add one of the following groups of ingredients—in the order listed—and cook for 5 more minutes, stirring frequently.

1. **BELL PEPPER MIX:** 1 tablespoon reduced-sodium soy sauce; 2 teaspoons sesame oil; ½ cup green or red bell pepper strips; ¼ medium onion, cut lengthwise into strips; ½ teaspoon red-pepper flakes

2. **VEGGIE BLEND:** 1 tablespoon hoisin sauce; 2 teaspoons sesame oil; ⅓ cup matchstick carrots; ⅓ cup chopped celery; 1 scallion, sliced; 2 tablespoons chopped unsalted peanuts

3. **ASPARAGUS AND CASHEW:** 1 tablespoon reduced-sodium soy sauce, 2 teaspoons sesame oil, ½ cup asparagus tips, 2 tablespoons chopped unsalted cashews

4. **SWEET LEMON:** 1 tablespoon reduced-sodium soy sauce; 1 tablespoon lemon juice; 1 teaspoon lemon peel; 1 teaspoon honey; 1 clove garlic, crushed; ½ cup snow peas; 1 cup chopped celery

5. **ASIAN BROCCOLI:** 1 whisked egg; ½ cup (or more) chopped broccoli; ¼ medium onion, cut lengthwise

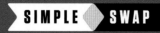

**SIMPLE SWAP**

Sesame oil gives stir-fries a distinct flavor. Nutritionally, it's similar to olive oil because it's full of heart-healthy unsaturated fat. (Make sure you get plain, not toasted, sesame oil.)

into long strips; ½ teaspoon red pepper flakes; 1 tablespoon reduced-sodium soy sauce

6. **HOISIN SNOW PEAS:** 1 whisked egg; ½ cup snow peas; ½ cup green or red bell pepper strips; ¼ onion, cut lengthwise into long strips; 1 tablespoon hoisin sauce

## GET BAKED

Preheat the oven to 350°F and douse your chicken in sauce, rub it with spices, crust it with goodies, or stuff it with savories. Bake uncovered for 20 to 25 minutes.

### SAUCES

*Watery baths like salsa will do just fine in the oven. But thicker sauces, like barbecue or ranch, must be mixed with water or broth or you'll be left with sticky, blackened char. Use a small baking dish with raised sides to keep the meat swimming.*

7. **FIESTA:** ⅓ cup salsa

8. **MELTED FIESTA:** 2 tablespoons jalapeño cheese dip, 2 tablespoons salsa, 1 tablespoon water

9. **ITALIAN:** 2 tablespoons marinara sauce, 2 tablespoons water

10. **TEXAS STYLE:** 2 tablespoons barbecue sauce, 2 tablespoons water

11. **RANCH DIPPED:** 2 tablespoons ranch dressing, 2 tablespoons water

12. **HONEY MUSTARD:** 2 tablespoons Dijon mustard, 2 tablespoons honey, 1 teaspoon olive oil

13. **SPICED UP:** 3 tablespoons chicken broth; 1 tablespoon mustard; 1 clove garlic, crushed

14. **CREAM OF MUSHROOM:** 2 tablespoons condensed mushroom soup, 2 tablespoons water

15. **PESTO:** 2 tablespoons pesto, 2 tablespoons reduced-sodium chicken broth

**16. SWEET AND SOUR:** 2 tablespoons reduced-sodium soy sauce, ¼ cup crushed pineapple with juice

 **2-SECOND LIFE CHANGER**

To lock in juices, sear the breast in a hot skillet for 1 to 2 minutes per side before baking.

**17. COCONUT CURRY:** 3 tablespoons chicken broth, 2 tablespoons light coconut milk, ¼ teaspoon curry powder

**18. APPLE GLAZE:** ⅓ cup chicken broth, 1 tablespoon maple syrup, 1 tablespoon apple juice

**19. BBQ SAUCE:** 3 tablespoons red wine vinegar; 1 tablespoon barbecue sauce; 1 clove garlic, crushed

**20. HOT STUFF:** 2 tablespoons hot sauce, 2 tablespoons Worcestershire sauce, ¼ teaspoon chili powder

**21. HERBED CITRUS:** 2 tablespoons lemon juice, 2 tablespoons orange marmalade, ¼ teaspoon rosemary

### RUBS

*Rub these mixtures evenly over each breast, then coat with cooking spray.*

**22. CHILI COVERED:** ¼ teaspoon each garlic powder, chili powder, black pepper, and oregano; salt to taste

**23. THREE-ALARM FIRE:** ¼ teaspoon each black pepper, chili powder, red-pepper flakes, cumin, and hot sauce

**24. TRI-HERB RUB:** ¼ teaspoon each dried basil, rosemary, and thyme; salt and pepper to taste

### CRUSTS

*Crack an egg into a shallow bowl, whisk it, dip the chicken in it, and then roll the chicken in a plate of one of these coatings.*

25. **NUT COVERED:** $\frac{1}{3}$ cup finely chopped nuts

26. **ITALIAN TOPPED:** 1 tablespoon finely grated Parmesan cheese, 1 tablespoon Italian bread crumbs, a pinch of black pepper

27. **FAUX FRIED:** $\frac{1}{2}$ cup crushed corn or bran flakes, or panko bread crumbs

*STUFFINGS*

*Pound the daylights out of your chicken breast with a meat tenderizer until it's uniformly thin. Then arrange any of the following ingredients on the breast, roll it up, and secure it with toothpicks or kitchen twine.*

28. **HAM AND CHEESE:** 1 slice Cheddar cheese, 2 slices deli ham, $\frac{1}{4}$ teaspoon black pepper

29. **STROMBOLI:** 1 slice mozzarella cheese; 3 slices pepperoni; 3 leaves fresh basil, chopped

30. **PIZZA:** 1 slice mozzarella; $\frac{1}{4}$ cup chopped tomatoes; 3 leaves fresh basil, chopped

31. **SPINACH STUFFED:** 1 small handful baby spinach leaves, chopped; 1 tablespoon blue-cheese crumbles; 1 clove garlic, crushed

32. **DELI STYLE:** 1 slice mozzarella, 1 slice salami, 1 tablespoon chopped roasted red pepper

33. **SUN-DRIED TOMATO:** $1\frac{1}{2}$ tablespoons part-skim ricotta cheese, 1 tablespoon chopped sun-dried tomatoes, $\frac{1}{4}$ teaspoon oregano

34. **MEDITERRANEAN:** $1\frac{1}{2}$ tablespoons part-skim ricotta cheese, 1 tablespoon finely chopped olives, $\frac{1}{4}$ teaspoon lemon peel

35. **PARMESAN PESTO:** 1 tablespoon pesto, 1 tablespoon shredded Parmesan cheese, $\frac{1}{4}$ teaspoon black pepper

## GRILL POWER

Soak the chicken in these marinades for at least an hour. Mix marinade ingredients well in a resealable plastic bag, drop in the chicken, seal, shake, and refrigerate. Heat a grill or place a nonstick skillet over medium-high heat on the stove. Cook for 3 to 5 minutes per side.

**36. BOOZE INFUSED:** 2 tablespoons bourbon, 1 teaspoon deli-style mustard, ¼ teaspoon black pepper

**37. SWEET BOOZE INFUSED:** 2 tablespoons bourbon; 1 teaspoon honey; 1 clove garlic, crushed

**38. RED WINE DRESSED:** 2 tablespoons red wine; 1 teaspoon barbecue sauce; 1 clove garlic, crushed

**39. WHITE WINE DRESSED:** 2 tablespoons white wine; 1 clove garlic, crushed; ¼ teaspoon thyme

**40. RICH AND CREAMY:** 2 tablespoons plain yogurt, ¼ teaspoon dill

**41. CURRY CREAM:** 2 tablespoons plain yogurt, 1 teaspoon olive oil, ¼ teaspoon curry powder

**42. MARGARITAVILLE:** 2 tablespoons lime juice, 1 teaspoon olive oil, ¼ teaspoon cilantro

**43. CUMIN AND LIME:** 2 tablespoons lime juice, ¼ teaspoon cumin, ¼ teaspoon red-pepper flakes

**44. LEMON ZEST:** 2 tablespoons lemon juice, ¼ teaspoon lemon peel, ¼ teaspoon black pepper

**45. BALSAMIC HERB:** 2 tablespoons vinaigrette, ¼ teaspoon rosemary

**46. GINGER SPICED:** 2 tablespoons orange juice, ¼ teaspoon ginger powder, ¼ teaspoon cilantro

**47. O-JUICED:** 2 tablespoons orange juice, 1 tablespoon hoisin sauce, ¼ teaspoon red-pepper flakes

**48. SODA POPPED:** 2 tablespoons cola, ¼ teaspoon black pepper

**49. RED-PEPPER POP:** 1 tablespoon reduced-sodium soy sauce, 1 teaspoon sesame oil, ¼ teaspoon red-pepper flakes

**50. HAWAIIAN PUNCH:** 2 tablespoons pineapple juice; 1 clove garlic, crushed; ¼ teaspoon black pepper

# INDIVIDUAL PIZZAS WITH GRUYÈRE, CARAMELIZED ONIONS, AND APPLES

4 teaspoons extra-virgin olive oil, divided
2 medium onions, halved and thinly sliced
¾ cup + 3 tablespoons water
2 medium red apples, halved, cored, and thinly sliced
2 cans (15 ounces each) cannellini beans, drained and rinsed
2 tablespoons fresh lemon juice
½ teaspoon salt
¼ teaspoon dried rosemary, crumbled
4 whole wheat tortillas (8″ diameter)
2 cups (8 ounces) shredded reduced-fat Gruyère cheese (or reduced-fat Swiss)
¼ cup chopped pecans

*Preheat the oven to 450°F. In a large skillet, warm 2 teaspoons of the oil over medium heat. Add the onions and toss to coat. Add ¾ cup water, bring to a boil, and cook 5 minutes longer. Add the apples. Cook the mixture until the apples are crisp-tender, onions are golden, and liquid has evaporated, 7 to 10 minutes. Meanwhile, in a medium bowl, mash the beans with the lemon juice, salt, rosemary, 3 tablespoons water, and the remaining 2 teaspoons oil.*

*Place the tortillas on 2 large baking sheets. Spread the beans evenly over the tortillas. Top with the onion-apple mixture, cheese, and pecans. Bake about 5 minutes, until the pizzas are piping hot and the cheese has melted. Serve hot.*

MAKES 4 PIZZAS: PER PIZZA: 648 CALORIES, 36 G PROTEIN, 78 G CARBOHYDRATES, 24 G TOTAL FAT, 7 G SATURATED FAT, 14 G FIBER, 844 MG SODIUM

LEFTOVER LOVE

COOKING FOR ONE? STORE THE EXTRA BEANS AND ONION-APPLE MIXTURE SEPARATELY (LET THE LATTER COOL COMPLETELY) IN THE REFRIGERATOR FOR A READY-TO-BUILD, NO-PREP PIZZA ANY NIGHT.

# Quick, Low-Fat Side Dishes

## SPICY CHARRED CAULIFLOWER

1 tablespoon ground cumin

1 tablespoon paprika

1 teaspoon garlic powder

1 teaspoon salt (+ additional to taste)

1 teaspoon black pepper (+ additional to taste)

2 heads cauliflower, sliced into 2 to 4 planks (slices) per head

Olive oil

*Preheat the oven to 500°F. Combine the spices, salt, and pepper and set aside. Brush the cauliflower planks on both sides with oil,* *season with additional salt and pepper, and lay on a baking sheet. Roast for 6 to 8 minutes or until the ends soften. Preheat a grill to medium. Brush a fresh layer of olive oil onto the cauliflower and sprinkle with the spice mix. Place each plank directly on the grill rack and cook until lightly charred, about 5 to 8 minutes. Flip and lightly char the other side.*

MAKES 4 SERVINGS. PER SERVING: 90 CALORIES, 6 G PROTEIN, 17 G CARBOHYDRATES, 2 G TOTAL FAT, 0 G SATURATED FAT, 7 G FIBER, 670 MG SODIUM

 **2-SECOND LIFE CHANGER**

The two biggest mistakes people make when microwaving vegetables are dousing them with too much water and cooking them way too long. Washing veggies and not drying them will add just enough water. Place them in a microwaveable dish with the lid slightly ajar—this will steam the veggies, yet let enough hot air escape to keep your side from exploding. As for cooking times, a good starting point is 1 minute for every cup of tender produce, like fresh spinach and asparagus, and 3 minutes for every cup of heartier fresh vegetables, such as broccoli and carrots. After the initial time is up, hit the "add 30 seconds" button until your veggies are the way you like them.

# SWEET POTATO FRIES

*Peel and cut 2 medium sweet potatoes into 12 equal wedges. Place them on a large baking sheet and toss with ½ tablespoon olive oil, adding salt, pepper, and ground red pepper to taste. Spread in an even layer and bake at 425°F until lightly browned and crisp to the touch. The natural sugars found within these fiber-packed spuds pair perfectly with the fiery ground red pepper. These fries are every bit as enjoyable as the ones fried up in restaurants across the country—for a fraction of the calories.*

MAKES 4 SERVINGS. PER SERVING: 70 CALORIES, 2 G TOTAL FAT, 0 G SATURATED FAT, 200 MG SODIUM

# SAUTÉED BRUSSELS SPROUTS

*Halve the sprouts and cook in a large skillet (don't crowd them!) with olive oil and chopped garlic. When tender, add 1 cup peeled, cubed apple pieces and a handful of pine nuts. Sauté for another few minutes and season with salt and pepper.*

PER SERVING (1 CUP COOKED): 55 CALORIES, 11 G CARBOHYDRATES, 1 G TOTAL FAT, 200 MG SODIUM

# PARMESAN ASPARAGUS

*Preheat the oven to 400°F. Lightly coat the spears with olive oil, salt and pepper, and a good grating of Parmesan cheese. Lay them out on a baking sheet and roast until the spears turn tender and the cheese is lightly browned (about 12 minutes). Before serving, squeeze a lemon over the top.*

PER SERVING (4 SPEARS): 40 CALORIES, 7 G CARBOHYDRATES, 25 MG SODIUM

# SPICY CHICKPEAS

*Sauté 2 cloves of garlic and a few pinches of red-pepper flakes in olive oil until fragrant, then stir in canned, drained chickpeas and cook until heated through.*

PER SERVING (¼ CUP COOKED): 65 CALORIES, 11 G CARBOHYDRATES, 1 G TOTAL FAT, 100 MG SODIUM

# HIDE YOUR VEGGIES!

**Could the same trick** that got you to eat your peas when you were a kid help you lose weight now? Penn State researchers think so. When pureed vegetables were sneaked into three daily meals, study subjects ate nearly 360 fewer calories than when they were given the regular versions. (That could add up to a 3-pound loss in 1 month!) Break out your blender or food processor and make these swaps.

### PASTA SALAD

*Skip . . .*
½ cup mayo

*Add . . .*
½ cup roasted peppers, pureed

*Save . . .*
435 calories

### VEGGIE DIP

*Skip . . .*
¼ cup sour cream

*Add . . .*
½ cup spinach, cooked, strained, and pureed

*Save . . .*
79 calories

### BROWNIE MIX

*Skip . . .*
All oil

*Add . . .*
½ cup pureed beets and 1 can (15.5 ounces) black beans, pureed

*Save . . .*
469 calories

### CHOWDER

*Skip . . .*
1 cup cream

*Add . . .*
2 cups sweet corn, pureed

*Save . . .*
556 calories

## SAUTÉED SNOW PEAS

2 tablespoons extra-virgin olive oil
2 tablespoons minced garlic
2 tablespoons finely chopped ginger
4 cups snow peas, ends cut off
¼ cup vegetable broth
2 tablespoons finely chopped parsley

*Pour the oil into a large skillet over medium heat. When it starts to shimmer, add the garlic and ginger and stir for about 3 minutes. Add the snow peas and toss a few times to coat, then add the broth. Continue cooking, stirring occasionally, for about 3 more minutes. Add the parsley just before removing the vegetables. Use tongs to transfer the peas to a plate and serve immediately. Tip: Splash a little vegetable broth into the pan. Then, as the liquid boils off, the veggies will steam while they're cooking in the oil.*

MAKES 4 SERVINGS. PER SERVING: 110 CALORIES, 2 G PROTEIN, 6 G CARBOHYDRATES, 8 G TOTAL FAT, 1 G SATURATED FAT, 2 G FIBER, 55 MG SODIUM

*"Success means doing the best we can with what we have.*
*Success is the doing, not the getting; in the trying, not the triumph."*

—ZIG ZIGLAR

# Top it off

▶ Don't sweat your sides and snacks. Enjoy the extras without going overboard with these tips.

## SLIM PICKINGS

Fruits are a healthy snack, but some contain a lot of sugar and calories. These four won't pack on pounds.

### RASPBERRIES (64 CALORIES PER CUP)

While all berries are great sources of hunger-quelling fiber, raspberries have the most (1 cup has more than 4 slices of whole grain bread, and twice as much as 1 cup of blueberries).

*Squeeze more in:* Drop frozen berries into chilled brewed tea for a sweet iced tea without added sugar.

### GRAPEFRUIT (82 CALORIES PER MEDIUM GRAPEFRUIT)

In a study published in the *Journal of Medicinal Food*, obese adults who ate half a grapefruit before each of their three daily meals lost 3 more pounds over the course of 12 weeks than those who skipped the grapefruit appetizer.

*Squeeze more in:* Citrus is a great complement to soy sauce and other Asian flavors. Add grapefruit segments to a stir-fry once everything else is cooked, then stir gently and heat until just warmed. Or try grapefruit as a delicious low-cal dessert: Add a tiny bit of honey, sprinkle on some cardamom, and leave it under the broiler for 2 to 3 minutes.

### APPLES (95 CALORIES PER MEDIUM APPLE)

An apple a day may keep the chub away: A study in the journal *Appetite* found that people who ate an apple consumed 15 percent fewer calories afterward than those who didn't eat the fruit. The fiber in apples slows digestion, and a medium apple has 4 filling grams of it (most of it's in the skin, so don't peel it!).

*Squeeze more in:* Toss chopped apple, jicama, and celery with olive oil, lemon juice, and honey for a refreshing side salad with a touch of sweetness.

### BANANAS (105 CALORIES PER MEDIUM BANANA)

Research reveals that the yellow guys contain "resistant starch," a type of fiber that your body digests more slowly, which keeps blood sugar stable and leaves you feeling satisfied longer.

*Squeeze more in:* Slice a banana in half, then cover each piece with ½ tablespoon of your favorite nut butter and ½ tablespoon of cocoa powder. Wrap the pieces in waxed paper and freeze for 10 to 15 minutes for a yummy dessert. (Makes 2 servings.)

## THE LOWEST-HANGING FRUIT

Unsweetened frozen fruit and water-packed canned fruit are worthy stand-ins for fresh produce. If you're watching your waistline, watch out for dried fruit: The concentrated sugars up the calorie count, plus it's less filling, which makes it easier to overeat.

# Pop Secrets

Popcorn is actually an incredibly underrated snack food—when it's not drenched in butter and salt, that is. A generous 3-cup serving has fewer

# THE BAR EXAM

Packaged on-the-go bars certainly can be a convenient nutrient-packed snack, but if you're not careful, you could be unwrapping candy in disguise. Keep these criteria in mind when reading the label.

- ✓ Protein: For it to be considered a "protein bar," it needs at least 6 grams. Research gives the advantage to whey, a dairy-derived protein, when it comes to body sculpting.

- ✓ Carbohydrates: 35 grams or less total, with no more than 19 grams from sugar. Carbs are best from sources like whole grains and dried fruit.

- ✓ Fat: 8 grams or less, from sources like nuts, seeds, and peanut butter. Watch for saturated fats, such as palm oil.

- ✓ Fiber: Up to 5 grams. Most bars don't identify the type of fiber they contain, but many have some combo of insoluble and soluble fiber.

than 100 calories, as much fiber as a cup of cooked brown rice, and more of the healthful antioxidant substances called polyphenols than fruits and vegetables, according to recent research from the University of Scranton in Pennsylvania. Whether you're craving sweet or savory, you can turn homemade popcorn into a superstar snack with one of these six tasty renditions. In a pinch, use olive oil spray as a low-calorie way to get toppings to stick.

## SLIM-DOWN SECRET

Researchers discovered that those bits of popcorn that always get stuck in your teeth (called hulls) actually have the highest concentration of polyphenols and fiber.

*Each recipe serves one. Nutritional information based on air-popped popcorn.*

## ROSEMARY PARMESAN

*In a small bowl, drizzle 3 cups popped popcorn with 1 teaspoon olive oil. Sprinkle with 1 teaspoon finely chopped fresh rosemary and 1 tablespoon grated Parmesan cheese, then toss well to coat evenly. Top with black pepper.*

PER SERVING: 160 CALORIES, 5 G PROTEIN, 19 G CARBOHYDRATES, 7 G TOTAL FAT, 1.5 G SATURATED FAT, 4 G FIBER, 80 MG SODIUM

## PIÑA COLADA

*Melt 1 teaspoon extra-virgin coconut oil in a small skillet over low heat for about 15 seconds, or microwave on high in a small glass dish for 30 seconds. Place 3 cups popped popcorn in a small bowl and drizzle with oil. Sprinkle with 1 finely chopped ring of dried pineapple, 2 teaspoons sweetened coconut flakes, and ⅛ teaspoon salt, then toss well to coat evenly.*

PER SERVING: 220 CALORIES, 3 G PROTEIN, 42 G CARBOHYDRATES, 7 G TOTAL FAT, 5 G SATURATED FAT, 4 G FIBER, 310 MG SODIUM

# CURRY CHIPOTLE

*In a small skillet, heat 1½ teaspoons canola oil, ½ teaspoon curry powder, ¼ teaspoon ground chipotle or chili powder, and ⅛ teaspoon salt over a low flame and whisk gently for 1 to 2 minutes, until the oil begins to bubble. Drizzle onto 3 cups popped popcorn in a small bowl, then toss well to coat evenly.*

PER SERVING: 160 CALORIES, 3 G PROTEIN, 20 G CARBOHYDRATES, 8 G TOTAL FAT, 0.5 G SATURATED FAT, 4 G FIBER, 290 MG SODIUM

# LEMON DILL

*Place 3 cups popped popcorn in a small bowl and drizzle with 1 teaspoon olive oil. Sprinkle with 1 teaspoon oregano, ½ teaspoon each dill and lemon peel, and ⅛ teaspoon salt, then toss well to coat.*

PER SERVING: 140 CALORIES, 3 G PROTEIN, 20 G CARBOHYDRATES, 6 G TOTAL FAT, 1 G SATURATED FAT, 4 G FIBER, 290 MG SODIUM

# SUGAR 'N' SPICE

*In a small bowl, drizzle 3 cups popped popcorn with 1 teaspoon flaxseed oil. Sprinkle with 1 teaspoon confectioners' sugar, ½ teaspoon ground cinnamon, ¼ teaspoon ground nutmeg, and ⅛ teaspoon salt, then toss well to coat evenly.*

PER SERVING: 150 CALORIES, 3 G PROTEIN, 23 G CARBOHYDRATES, 6 G TOTAL FAT, 0.5 G SATURATED FAT, 4 G FIBER, 290 MG SODIUM

# CRAN-CHOCOLATE

*In a small glass bowl, microwave 1 tablespoon dark chocolate chips until just beginning to melt (about 45 seconds). Mix well with a rubber spatula until chocolate is about three-quarters of the way melted; some lumps should remain. Put 3 cups popped popcorn in a medium bowl and top with the melted chocolate. Sprinkle with 2 tablespoons dried cranberries and ⅛ teaspoon salt, then mix thoroughly. Place the bowl in the refrigerator for 10 minutes to harden the chocolate.*

PER SERVING: 210 CALORIES, 4 G PROTEIN, 38 G CARBOHYDRATES, 6 G TOTAL FAT, 3 G SATURATED FAT, 5 G FIBER, 290 MG SODIUM

# JIFFY POPPED

The way you pop your kernels can quickly put a dent in their healthful image. Here's how three cooking methods compare.

### AIR POPPER

A popper will cost at least $15 and take up cabinet space, but it uses no oil—and adds no calories.

*DO IT:*
Follow the machine's instructions!

### STOVE TOP

Popcorn is very crisp and has rich flavor, but the oil adds about 70 calories.

*DO IT:*
Add a scant 2 teaspoons of peanut or canola oil to a heavy-bottom pot over medium-high heat. When the oil is hot, add 1½ heaping tablespoons of kernels. Replacethe lid and gently shake the pot to heat evenly. When the popping slows after 2 to 3 minutes, turn off the heat. Wait 30 seconds before removing the lid to allow kernels to finish popping. Makes about 3 cups.

### MICROWAVE

The fluffiness of each kernel will depend on the microwave's wattage, but cleanup is minimal—you can cook, top, and serve your snack in the same bowl.

*DO IT:*
Add 1½ heaping tablespoons of kernels to a tempered-glass microwave-safe bowl with a vented lid. Cook on high for 2 to 3 minutes. The bowl will be hot, so use oven mitts. Makes about 3 cups popped popcorn.

# Skinny Dips

Dips don't really have a rep for raising the nutritional value of whatever you're pairing them with. More often than not, they just pack on calories. But I find something so satisfying about bringing an appetizer to a party that's so rich and delicious that no one knows it's healthy. (It started with making over my favorite, buffalo chicken dip.) Impress your friends with one of these seven healthy alternatives that still pack plenty of taste.

## EDAMAME HUMMUS

1 cup frozen shelled edamame
1 teaspoon chopped garlic
1 tablespoon tahini
1 tablespoon fresh lemon juice
3 tablespoons water
¼ teaspoon salt
1 tablespoon olive oil
½ teaspoon Sriracha (optional)

*Boil the edamame for 4 to 6 minutes, then drain. Combine in a food processor with the garlic, tahini, lemon juice, water, and salt and blend well. Drizzle in the olive oil. Process until smooth. (If the texture is too thick, add another tablespoon of water.)*

MAKES 4 SERVINGS. PER SERVING: 101 CALORIES, 5 G PROTEIN, 5 G CARBOHYDRATES, 7 G TOTAL FAT, 2 G FIBER, 152 MG SODIUM

LIGHTER BITE

## KALE CHIPS FOUR WAYS

CHOP A BUNCH OF DRY KALE LEAVES (DINOSAUR KALE, CURLY KALE, OR A MIXTURE), DRIZZLE WITH OLIVE OIL, SPRINKLE WITH ONE OF THE SEASONINGS BELOW, AND TOSS; PLACE ON A BAKING SHEET AND BAKE AT 325°F UNTIL CRISPY, OR ABOUT 20 TO 35 MINUTES.

| Lemon peel and sea salt | Paprika, chipotle pepper, and sea salt | Roasted sesame oil, roasted sesame seeds, and sea salt | Shredded white Cheddar cheese, fresh ground black pepper |
|---|---|---|---|

# TROPICAL GUAC

½ avocado, pitted, peeled, and chopped
⅛ teaspoon salt
2 tablespoons chopped red onion
1½ tablespoons chopped fresh cilantro
2 teaspoons chopped jalapeño chile pepper
2 teaspoons fresh lime juice
¼ cup chopped pineapple
¼ cup chopped mango
¼ cup chopped cantaloupe

*Mash the avocado and salt together with a fork. Gently stir in the onion, cilantro, jalapeño, and lime juice. Fold in the pineapple, mango, and cantaloupe.*

MAKES 4 SERVINGS. PER SERVING: 107 CALORIES, 2 G PROTEIN, 19 G CARBOHYDRATES, 4 G TOTAL FAT, 4 G FIBER, 88 MG SODIUM

---

# COOL CUCUMBER-HERB DIP

1 tablespoon finely chopped shallot
½ cup chopped cucumber, seeds removed
1 cup low-fat sour cream
1 teaspoon white wine vinegar
1 tablespoon chopped fresh dill
1 tablespoon chopped fresh chives
¼ teaspoon salt
Freshly ground black pepper

*In a food processor, combine the shallot and cucumber; discard the extra liquid. In a separate bowl, mix the sour cream with the shallot-cucumber mixture. Stir in the vinegar, dill, chives, and salt, then add the pepper to taste. Refrigerate up to 2 hours to allow flavors to develop.*

MAKES 4 SERVINGS. PER SERVING: 82 CALORIES, 2 G PROTEIN, 5 G CARBOHYDRATES, 6 G TOTAL FAT, 4 G SATURATED FAT, 186 MG SODIUM

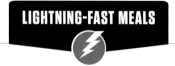

## LIGHTNING-FAST MEALS

### ONE-STEP HOMEMADE HUMMUS:

In a food processor, combine 1 clove garlic (chopped), a 15-ounce can of chickpeas (drained and rinsed), 2 tablespoons each tahini, lemon juice, extra-virgin olive oil, and water, and ½ teaspoon each ground cumin and salt; blend until smooth. You'll get 2 cups of dip that will keep for a week in the fridge.

# SWEET-AND-SPICY YOGURT

1 cup low-fat plain Greek yogurt
2 tablespoons finely chopped ripe peach
1 teaspoon lemon juice
1 dash Worcestershire sauce
1½ teaspoons curry powder
¼ teaspoon ground cumin
¼ teaspoon salt

*In a bowl, stir together all the ingredients. Chill up to 2 hours to allow the flavors to develop. Top with chopped red bell pepper and scallion for garnish.*

MAKES 4 SERVINGS. PER SERVING: 42 CALORIES, 5 G PROTEIN, 3 G CARBOHYDRATES, 1 G TOTAL FAT, 165 MG SODIUM

# CHEESY TOMATO DIP

1 tomato, quartered, seeds removed
6 ounces feta cheese, crumbled
1 teaspoon lemon juice
⅛ teaspoon dried oregano
1 tablespoon chopped kalamata olives
1 tablespoon chopped sun-dried tomatoes
(packed in oil, drained)

*In a food processor, chop the tomato. Add the feta in small batches, blending to combine. Pour in the lemon juice and oregano and blend again. In a bowl, fold the olives into the cheese-tomato mixture. Top with the sun-dried tomatoes.*

MAKES 4 SERVINGS. PER SERVING: 122 CALORIES, 6 G PROTEIN, 3 G CARBOHYDRATES, 9 G TOTAL FAT, 6 G SATURATED FAT, 495 MG SODIUM

# SWEET DESSERT DELIGHT

½ cup + 2 tablespoons frozen blueberries
(thawed)
4 ounces low-fat ricotta
2 tablespoons orange juice
1 teaspoon vanilla
2 teaspoons honey
½ teaspoon ground cinnamon

*In a food processor, combine all the ingredients and blend until smooth. Chill in the refrigerator. Serve with fruit, graham crackers, or cinnamon twists. Don't have time to thaw the blueberries? Pop them in the microwave until just warmed through (about 40 seconds).*

MAKES 4 SERVINGS. PER SERVING: 68 CALORIES, 3 G PROTEIN, 9 G CARBOHYDRATES, 2 G TOTAL FAT, 1 G SATURATED FAT, 35 MG SODIUM

# SLAM DUNKS!

**Ditch the boring veggies** and give pita chips a break—try one of these creative low-cal swaps instead.

| | | |
|---|---|---|
| **ENDIVE** | **SWEET POTATOES** | **SUMMER SQUASH** |
| Put a dab of dip in the center of a boat-shaped leaf and roll it up. | Cut the spuds into wedges and give them the same treatment as okra. | Slice into rounds or matchsticks, then dust lightly with salt. |
| **OKRA** | **SHRIMP** | **SUGAR SNAP PEAS** |
| Season with olive oil, salt, and pepper, then roast at 400°F for 20 minutes. | Boil with a little Old Bay seasoning and lemon juice. | Eat them raw. They're crunchy, low-cal (just 14 calories per 10 pods), and full of vitamin C. |

*"Don't wait
until you
reach your goal
to be
proud of yourself.
Be proud of yourself
every step
of the way."*

—UNKNOWN

# INDEX

**Boldface** page references indicate photographs. <u>Underscored</u> references indicate boxed text.

Step up with knee drive, 119, **119**
Step up workout, 174–77, **174–77**
Stir-fry, chicken recipes, 305–6
Straight-leg deadlifts, 80, **80**
Straight-leg dumbbell deadlift, 127, **127**
Strength increase from short workouts, 8
Strength training
  calories burned by, 70–71, 83
  circuit training, 70
  exercise machine replacement exercises, 75–78, **75–78**
  for fast weight loss
    5 pounds, 221–22
    10 pounds, 220–21
    20+ pounds, 219
  grip, 81, 81
  intensity increase with explosive movements, 89
  functional training, 86–87
  heavier weights, 85
  intervals (Tabata method), 88
  less rest between moves, 87, 87–89
  tempo, 82–84
  losing your fear of lifting, 70
  muscle building with, 73
  myths, 70–73
  number of repetitions, 85
  selective, 93–94, 94
  speed of lifting, 82–84, 83
  starting weights for beginners, 84
Stress
  physical reaction to, 248
  stress busters, 249–50
Stretching, 205
Sugar, average daily consumption of, 55
Sumo squat with lateral raise, 133, **133**
Supermarket survival guide, 25–27

Supersets, 87, 87
Support of friends and family, 229, 229–30
Suspended biceps curls, 164, **164**
Suspended chest press, 163, **163**
Suspended overhead triceps extensions, 164, **164**
Suspended power pull, 164, **164**
Suspended pushup, 108, **108**
Suspended row, 112, **112**, 163, **163**
Suspended squat jumps, 163, **163**
Swearing, as stress buster, 249
Sweating, 38
Sweet potato fries, 312
Swimming, 211–12, 213

# T

Tabata method, 88
Talk test, 199
Tempo, lifting, 82–84, 83, 225
Tempos (cardio intervals), 196, 203–4, 221
Tendonitis, 235
Tennis elbow, 235
Thighs, foam roller exercise for, 191, **191**
Thinking sharper, with exercise, 232
Tight core rotations, 66, **66**
Toe raises, 101
Tomato
  canned whole peeled, 31
  Cheesy Tomato Dip, 323
  preparation for cooking, 39
Total-body training (burpee) workout, 139–44, **140–43**
Trans fats, 19
TRX, 92, 162–64
Turkey
  Herb-Roasted Turkey Breast, 303
  Turkey Burger, 291

# U

Underhand grip, **81**, 81
Upside-down snow angel, 188, **188**

# V

Valslide arm circle, 188, **188**
Valslide curtsy lunge, 186, **186**
Valslide pike, 186, **186**
Valslide pushup, 187, **187**
Valslides, 91, 109
Valslide workout, 185–88, **186–88**
Vegetables
  cooking techniques, 34–38
  hiding, 313
  microwaving, 311
  preparation for cooking, 39
  side dishes, 311–14
Vinaigrettes, 278, 278–79, 279
Vinegar, balsamic, 31

# W

Waist circumference, activity level and, 3
Walking lunge, 111, **111**
Warmup, 65–69
Washing dishes, posture for, 259
Water, 41, 227, 251, 251–52
Weigh-ins, frequent, 218
Weight cycling, 11–13
Weight gain, with irregular exercise pattern, 12–13
Weight increase, technological advances and, 4
Weight lifting. See Strength training
Weight loss. See also Fat loss
  fastest methods for
    5 pounds, 221–22
    10 pounds, 220–21
    20+ pounds, 219–20